T0306156

Learning from Clinical Cases in Primary Care

This new book is designed around 20 clinical cases, each representative of scenarios encountered by doctors who work in primary care and which will prompt learning in related issues surrounding each clinical scenario. Each case description concludes with an initial exam style question, which Membership of the Royal College of General Practitioners (MRCGP) candidates will recognize as being directed towards learning for the Applied Knowledge Test (AKT). An expanded answer to that initial question is followed by a detailed explanation, concluding with further questions for self-assessment and reflection.

The cases also provide a template for the preparation of the Simulated Consultation Assessment (SCA) component of the MRCGP exam and can be used by trainers and trainees alike as a prototype for role play. Some cases offer learning opportunities through discussion of discrete clinical entities, whilst others use the clinical cases to introduce the reader to broader concepts that often need grappling with in primary care.

Covering the wide range of specialities that are encountered in primary care, the book reflects the remarkable breadth of clinical knowledge that is required of a primary care practitioner and demonstrates why general practice remains a challenging but rewarding specialty to master.

Learning from Clinical Cases in Primary Care

For MRCGP and Beyond

Samar Razaq
MBChB, MRCGP, DGM, DCH, DRCOG
General Practitioner
Buckinghamshire, UK

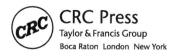

CRC Press
Taylor & Francis Group
Boca Raton London New York

CRC Press is an imprint of the
Taylor & Francis Group, an **informa** business

Designed cover image: Credit: sturti. Getty Images.

First edition published 2025
by CRC Press
2385 NW Executive Center Drive, Suite 320, Boca Raton, FL 33431

and by CRC Press
4 Park Square, Milton Park, Abingdon, Oxon, OX14 4RN

CRC Press is an imprint of Taylor & Francis Group, LLC

© 2025 Samar Razaq

ISBN: 9781032583570 (hbk)
ISBN: 9781032577203 (pbk)
ISBN: 9781003449737 (ebk)

DOI: 10.1201/9781003449737

Typeset in Minion
by Deanta Global Publishing Services, Chennai, India

Contents

Introduction

HOW TO USE THIS BOOK

Medicine, over the last two centuries, has made astounding progress. The remarkable feats of vaccination, anaesthesia, diagnostic imaging, drug development and gene therapy (amongst countless other accomplishments) are well known and well documented. However, in all this time, the art of medicine has perhaps remained unchanged. For the vast majority of contacts with patients, the practice of medicine does not rely on the dizzying array of complicated tests and procedures. It continues to hinge around a comprehensive history and a meticulous examination, aided by simple supplementary investigations when indicated. Amongst all the disciplines of medicine, this is probably most apparent in primary care. Whilst our hospital colleagues delineate the anatomy of patients with magnetic resonance imaging (MRI) scans, cure leukaemia with base edited T cells and measure blood pressure with arterial lines, the GP trundles along with their stethoscope (invented 1816) and blood pressure machine (invented in the 1800s) on a home visit in the hope of curing and reassuring their elderly patient. However, arguably, it is here that the art of medicine is practised at its finest.

The manner and setting in which disease and illness present to a GP are different from how they may present to other specialities. The punctuation of the time-tested consultation process in primary care with the fabulous advancements of modern medicine is the exception rather than the norm. Yet, it remains the arena in which the greatest number of patient contacts take place and majority of medical issues are suspected, managed and resolved. This uniqueness lends some differences to the primary care consultation when compared with other specialties, which I hope to shed some light on in the remaining introduction below.

A 74-year-old smoker presents clutching his chest, finding it difficult to breathe. He complains of a two-hour history of chest tightness, with pain radiating down his left arm and into the neck. He feels nauseous with the pain and feels that he may die very soon.

Not many would argue that the most likely diagnosis here is a myocardial infarction (MI), and calling for an ambulance is in urgent demand here, if the patient is not already in casualty. This classical presentation of an MI is the most commonly taught in medical textbooks but is largely irrelevant in primary care. Many primary care physicians will have diagnosed MIs, but few will have presented in this fashion to their surgeries. In my years of practising, I have not seen an MI present in this way in the community. In actual fact, if all MIs did present this way, it would make life a lot easier. This is, perhaps, the more likely way that an MI may present to casualty.

Now consider this scenario:

A 68-year-old non-smoker, with a strong family history of ischaemic heart disease, complains of feeling tired for the last three days. He has been having a feeling of indigestion and bloating in the epigastric area for the same period of time. He feels tight in his upper abdomen. He doesn't feel short of breath, but increased activity makes him feel nauseous. He has been taking over-the-counter indigestion medication to little avail. Examination is unremarkable, and he looks well whilst seated in the surgery. He is prescribed a course of proton pump inhibitors and asked to have a precautionary electrocardiogram (ECG) later that morning along with some blood tests. The hospital laboratory calls later in the afternoon to inform you that the patient has a troponin level 10 times above normal.

The late afternoon scramble that generally ensues is not likely to be too unfamiliar to many GPs.

In another scenario, the 68 year old may present to casualty an hour after seeing the GP, in the same manner as the 74 year old in the first scenario. He may feel aggrieved that he only saw his GP an hour ago, who was unable to diagnose him correctly. Unfortunately, it is not too uncommon for the casualty doctor to sympathize with the patient, ignoring basic dynamics in how disease may present in primary care.

FORMAT OF THE BOOK

The book, as the title suggests, is designed to encourage learning through clinical cases such as those discussed above. The 20 cases included in Section 1 will be familiar to doctors who work in primary care and will prompt learning in issues surrounding each clinical scenario. Each case is followed by an extended answer, concluding with exam style questions, which MRCGP hopefuls will recognize as being directed towards learning for the Applied Knowledge Test (AKT). Answers to these questions can be found at the end of the cases in Section 2. The case itself provides a template for the preparation of the Simulated Consultation Assessment (SCA) component of the MRCGP exam. It can be used by trainers and trainees alike as a prototype for role play. Some cases offer learning opportunities through discussion of discrete clinical entities, whilst others use the clinical cases to introduce the reader to concepts that often need grappling with in primary care.

The text is interspersed with bullet points and important tips to aid the learning process and encourage reader reflection. Each case is then followed by further multiple choice, single best answer and extended matching questions, which will help expand knowledge around loosely connected topics and provide further invaluable preparation for the AKT.

The cases and the explanation around them, like a typical GP clinic, can never be exhaustive. The book can only ever hope to be a small jigsaw piece of a much larger puzzle, which represents the practice of medicine. However, I hope that it will cover a wide range of specialties that are encountered in primary care and help the reader prepare for their exams and the trainers guide their trainees. But above all, I hope it will demonstrate the remarkable breadth of clinical knowledge that is required of a primary care practitioner and demonstrate why general practice remains an exceptionally difficult specialty to master.

SECTION 1

CASES

Case 1: The metamorphosis of disease presentation

An 80-year-old woman is seen during a home visit with 24 hours of left buttock pain. She had been involved with some birthday celebrations the day before, but this felt slightly different from her usual musculoskeletal pain. She is found well, fully mobile and comfortable in the house. No restriction in movement is noted. All her observations are normal, and she provides a urine sample, due to a history of renal colic, which is normal. Abdominal examination is performed as she feels the pain occasionally in her groin, and this is normal also. As she had not taken any analgesia, she is advised to take some painkillers and call back if the pain does not settle. Four hours later, she collapses and dies in casualty. Post-mortem reveals a ruptured abdominal aortic aneurysm (AAA).

Which of the following statements regarding AAA is false?

a. Computerized tomography (CT) scan is the most cost effective method for screening for an AAA.
b. Most AAAs are asymptomatic until rupture.
c. AAAs are more than four times more prevalent amongst smokers than in lifelong non-smokers.
d. The sensitivity of abdominal palpation for the detection of AAAs is inversely proportional to the size of the abdominal wall.
e. Rupture of the anterolateral wall of the aorta with bleeding into the peritoneum will often lead to immediate death.

DOI: 10.1201/9781003449737-2

ANSWER

a is false

It is perhaps apt to start the book with a case that probably represents the biggest challenge for the new and old general practitioner (GP) alike: dealing with uncertainty. One could successfully argue that the difference between an experienced GP and a new trainee is nothing other than their ability to successfully deal with the uncertainty that is inherent in the practice of primary care. The case will not delve into the peculiarities of the management of an AAA, but will rather concentrate on how this scenario demonstrates some important principles of the general practice consultation.

One of the challenges as a trainer is cultivating a balance in the new trainee between over-reacting to every symptom that the patient professes and not ignoring the gem hidden amongst all the distraction. New trainees, having recently completed undergraduate training and placements in hospital, may be used to having a set of signs and symptoms that conveniently point towards a diagnosis, thus making the process of decision making, in terms of management, easy. However, in general practice, a firm or concrete diagnosis is not always available. John Howie recognized this 50 years ago when he called "diagnosis" the Achilles' heel of general practice. Five decades later, we still find ourselves relying heavily on Voltaire's aphorism of *amusing the patient whilst nature cures the disease*. It may require multiple contacts with a GP before a firm diagnosis is made, if ever. Young doctors who have been brought up on a healthy dose of the definitiveness of a diagnosis associated with set management plans are likely to find this foray of general practice into the vague and inconcrete slightly disconcerting.

In the index case, things rapidly progressed with devastating consequences. Was there something about the consultation process that was responsible for this downturn of events? The consultation process between patient and doctor is a complex interplay of various factors, the ultimate aim being, simply put, problem resolution. The doctor and the patient, therefore, form the core of the interaction, with ideas, concerns and expectations being explored, modified and confronted, hopefully resulting in a harmonious agreement between the two parties. However, there is the obvious third component of the consultation: the presenting disease. Those who have practised medicine long enough will know that a disease may not always be present. However, this is not the starting assumption in most consultations, where an inquisitive mind assumes the presence of disease and works to either prove or disprove its existence. The way that disease presents will vary, but the most disconcerting aspect of its presentation is that it may be different to two physicians at two different times. As GPs, it is not unusual to face resistance from hospital doctors for a referral due to a lack of "hard" signs and symptoms, only for the original suspicions to be confirmed on hospital admission. Conversely, it is also not unusual to receive a somewhat disbelieving letter from casualty expressing amazement at how the GP could have missed the most obvious of conditions.

Consider Cases A and B below.

Case A. A 63-year-old woman has been seeing her GP for approximately 10 years for joint pains. After the first few visits, blood tests organized to rule out inflammatory disease were normal. A diagnosis of fibromyalgia is made, particularly since her symptoms became worse after the sudden death of her husband and the ensuing depression. A few years after the initial presentation, she develops swollen joints and pain again and has another battery of blood tests, which are negative. She is referred to the rheumatologist, who eventually confirms the diagnosis of fibromyalgia. Regular visits to the GP continue. In the 10th year of her initial presentation, rheumatoid arthritis is eventually diagnosed after the synovial swelling returns, coupled with a positive rheumatoid factor test. Disease-modifying anti-rheumatic drugs (DMARDs) are started, and all her symptoms resolve.

Case B. A 75-year-old woman attends with a three-day history of cough, wheeze, minimal amounts of productive mucus and mild shortness of breath. She complains of feeling hot and cold. A chest infection is diagnosed based on crepitations in the lung bases and the suggestive history. She returns two weeks later feeling slightly better but breathing still not having returned to normal and still having a fair bit of cough. She is noted to be well without any obvious shortness of breath, and a second course of antibiotics is prescribed on the assumption of a non-fully resolved infection. She returns two weeks later not feeling fully back to normal and having mild shortness of breath. This time, she mentions a mildly tender and swollen calf, which has become more noticeable over a few weeks. Blood oxygen saturation is at 96%. She is referred to hospital and eventually diagnosed with bilateral pleural emboli.

These cases demonstrate the well-known ambiguity of disease presentation. However, the cases differ in the time scale between what may be considered the start of the presentation and its final manifestation in a clinically recognizable form. Figure 1.1 aims to demonstrate this.

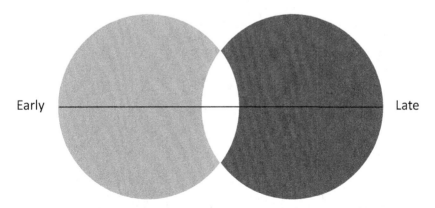

Early ——————————————————————————— Late

Gray - Vague symptomology
White - High index of suspicion required
Dark gray - Greatest diagnostic certainty

Figure 1.1   Manifestation of disease.

Whether one is able to make a successful diagnosis depends upon where along the continuum, expressed in Figure 1.1 as the timeline running through the diagram, the patient presents. In the green area, symptoms are likely to be vague, and examination and investigations may not yield meaningful results. In the dark gray area, the diagnosis may be obvious, with the patient presenting with "textbook" signs and symptoms and investigations pointing to a high probability of disease. Casualty physicians operate mainly in the dark gray area, with patients presenting late in the illness with classical symptoms. As GPs, we are often operating in the gray zone, an area of vague symptomology and sometimes aimless groping in the dark. Hence the importance of safety netting and constant review of patients in whom the symptoms fail to resolve or progress further. Worryingly, though, for GPs, the index case demonstrates that the best of safety netting may sometimes not be adequate: a serious, life-threatening condition masquerading as something benign, only for it to show its devastating effects in a matter of hours. The casualty physician who saw the same patient, whilst her presentation was in the dark gray zone, may well have pondered on how the GP who saw her only a few hours earlier managed to miss the diagnosis. It seems that this patient missed the white zone of Figure 1.1, or was unfortunately not attended to as she passed through it. Cases A and B, however, seem to have a definitive phase through this transformative form of the presentation when the illness briefly seems to mimic something clinically recognizable. A high index of suspicion is required at this stage to help make the diagnosis. It would be easy to miss this phase in patients who visit their doctor often, when it is all too easy to put down their symptoms to psychosomatic causes. Figure 1.2 aims to look at features of illnesses that should keep the physician on high alert.

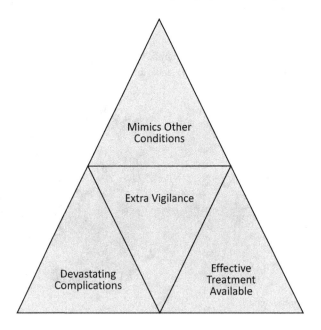

Figure 1.2 Triad of hypervigilance.

All of the above cases mimicked other conditions (fibromyalgia, chest infection, musculoskeletal back pain), can have devastating complications (joint deformity and death), and at least in Cases A and B, have effective treatments. If the discerning doctor is not on the lookout, the disease may well progress from white to dark gray (or beyond!), at which point unnecessary distress may result to the patient, and an uncomfortable confrontation may ensue.

Learning Tip

Stories are a great way of learning. Experienced GPs will be able to impart a huge amount of knowledge to trainee doctors just by recounting clinical encounters with patients. Stories are also used among colleagues to debrief and gauge the opinion of peers. These "stories" can impart useful clinical knowledge and convey the intricacies that are inherent in the management of clinically complex cases. It is surprising how much can be learnt by just discussing what happened, what one did in response and how that changed things. Stories give insights not only into clinical aspects of management but also into organizational obstacles that one may encounter. Unsurprisingly, this is recognized as an effective way of teaching and learning in clinical practice (see Cox in the Bibliography).

In summary, it is useful to consider the disease as a separate entity in the consultation process and be wary that it may take many forms before it lifts its veil to fully reveal itself. Whereas illness is often present, disease may lurk in and out of the GP consultation like a stealthy thief, only to be caught by the most attentive of detectives. We will now explore some of the concepts raised in this case that lead into the following case of Kawasaki disease.

AKT PREPARATION

Options for questions 1–5:

a. Eye test
b. Simple analgesia
c. Antihypertensive
d. MRI brain
e. Pizotifen
f. 100% Oxygen
g. Oral contraceptive pill
h. Blood pressure recording

For questions 1–5, choose the most appropriate management option from the list above. Each option may be used once, more than once or not at all.

1. A 12-year-old girl presents with a one-year history of periodic, pulsating, unilateral headache with no obvious trigger. The headache is preceded by flashes of light in the ipsilateral eye and is accompanied by nausea. The headache disappears with a combination of simple analgesia and lying down. Mum suffers from similar attacks. The frequency of headaches is now beginning to affect school. Neurological examination is normal.

2. A six-year-old boy presents with Mum, who reports a three-month history of intermittent frontal headache, which occasionally extends to behind the eyes. It is usually present in the latter part of the day and settles with simple analgesia or having a rest. The child is otherwise well.

3. A 15-year-old boy presents to casualty with a third episode of intense right-sided headache, which came on suddenly. He appears agitated and restless, and you find it difficult to perform an adequate neurological examination. His ipsilateral eye is red and watery and appears swollen. The last two episodes, which occurred in the last two weeks, lasted about an hour each.

4. Which of the following statements regarding Hodgkin's lymphoma are true?

    a. Lower socioeconomic groups are associated with a greater risk of developing Hodgkin's disease.
    b. Epstein–Barr virus infection has been implicated strongly in the development of Hodgkin's lymphoma.
    c. Reed–Sternberg cells are pathognomic of Hodgkin's lymphoma.
    d. The presence of B symptoms is associated with a worse prognosis.
    e. St Jude staging system is used to stage Hodgkin's lymphoma.

5. Deficiency of factor IX results in which inherited condition?

    a. Christmas disease
    b. Von Willebrand disease
    c. Haemophilia A
    d. Idiopathic thrombocytopaenic purpura (ITP)
    e. Bernard–Soulier syndrome

BIBLIOGRAPHY

Brown JK, Minns RA. Disorders of the central nervous system. In: Campbell AGM, McIntosh N. *Forfar & Arneil's Textbook of Pediatrics*. Churchill Livingstone; 1998. P. 641–846.

Cox K. Stories as case knowledge: Case knowledge as stories. *Med Educ* 2001; **35**(9):862–6.

Eden OB. Oncology and terminal care. In: Campbell AGM, McIntosh N. *Forfar & Arneil's Textbook of Pediatrics*. Churchill Livingstone; 1998. P. 884–933.

Gil-Gouveia R, Martins IP. Headaches associated with refractive errors: Myth or reality? *Headache* 2002 Apr; **42**(4):256–62.

Howie JG. Diagnosis: The Achilles heel? *J R Coll Gen Pract* 1972; **22**:310–15.

Majumdar A, Ahmed MA, Benton S. Cluster headache in children: Experience from a specialist headache clinic. *Eur J Paediatr Neurol* 2009 Nov; **13**(6):524–9.

Sakalihasan N, Limet R, Defawe OD. Abdominal aortic aneurysm. *Lancet* 2005 Apr 30–May 6; **365**(9470):1577–89.

Teleanu RI, Vladacenco O, Teleanu DM, Epure DA. Treatment of pediatric migraine: A review. *Maedica (Bucur)* 2016 Jun; **11**(2):136–43.

2

Case 2: Kawasaki disease

The last appointment in your morning emergency clinic is a three-year-old girl. Before you call her in, you decide to have a quick look at her notes and notice the following entries in chronological order over the last few days.

Day 1. 12-hour history of fever. Difficult to control with antipyretics. Reduced oral intake. On examination (o/e) appears well. T 38.5 °C. No rashes. No meningism. Ear nose and throat (ENT) and chest examination normal. Abdomen soft and non-tender. start of viral infection. Advised to observe, push fluids and review if any concerns.

Day 2. High fever continues. Now developed conjunctivitis and achy joints. O/e well hydrated. Inflamed conjunctiva. Pharynx inflamed. T 39.0 °C. No meningism. Tender anterior cervical lymph nodes. No joint swelling. ?—Streptococcal infection. Script for phenoxymethylpenicillin 125 mg/5 mL. 5 mL four times a day.

Day 3. Developed rash within few hours of starting penicillin so mum stopped medicine. O/e morbilliform rash on abdomen and chest. Mild scarlatiniform rash on arms and legs. Throat remains injected and conjunctiva slightly improved. ?—Scarlet fever. ?— Reaction to penicillin. Throat swab taken and treatment switched to erythromycin. To be continued for 10 days.

Today is day 5 of the illness. You have the throat swab results in front of you, which reads: *Throat swab: Normal upper respiratory tract flora.*

As you call the child in, you notice that the rash is still apparent on her body. Mum says the fever has persisted and she does not feel she is any better at all. You note that she has cracked lips, a swollen red tongue, high fever and mild oedema of her hands and feet.

Which of the following statements regarding Kawasaki disease is/are true?

a. Kawasaki disease is a self-limiting condition.
b. Kawasaki disease is most common in the first six months of life with a second peak in incidence after the sixth decade of life.
c. Management of the above child was inappropriate, as she fulfilled the criteria for the diagnosis of Kawasaki disease on day 3.
d. Effective treatment to prevent the coronary complications of Kawasaki disease is available.
e. Aspirin, during the febrile phase of the illness, is contraindicated in this child due to the risk of developing Reye's syndrome.

DOI: 10.1201/9781003449737-3

ANSWER

a and d are true

This case demonstrates how difficult it may be to make a correct diagnosis of a rare condition, particularly when it so often mimics much more commonly encountered conditions. Physicians should have a high index of suspicion and be extra vigilant of any rare condition that has the triad of features discussed in Case 1: mimics much commoner, less serious conditions, making diagnosis difficult; has devastating complications; and has effective treatment when diagnosed early (Figure 1.2). Bacterial meningitis fits the bill for this triad and is usually what most parents and health care workers are concerned about. However, Kawasaki disease is an important diagnosis that needs to be considered in any child with a persistent fever, as it, arguably, fulfils the aforementioned trio of features more aptly. Kawasaki disease is a self-limiting vasculitis that can occur in children of any age. It is more common in children between the ages of six months and five years. In the absence of treatment, symptoms and signs will normally resolve over the course of 10 days. The exact cause of Kawasaki disease remains elusive. Infectious agents are frequently suggested as the cause, based on the seasonal peaks of Kawasaki disease in various geographical regions. This is supported by the fact that it is uncommon in children under the age of three months, suggesting a protective role of transplacental antibodies against the infectious agent. Bacterial toxins behaving as superantigens and triggering off an inflammatory cascade have also been suggested but have never been convincingly isolated in patients with the condition. Incidence in the UK is estimated at eight cases per 100,000 in children under the age of five. Increased recognition of the condition is thought to be responsible for the rising incidence (Harnden et al.). Incidence is higher amongst Asians from the Indian subcontinent (Gardner-Medwin et al.).

Mimics other conditions: A diagnostic test for Kawasaki disease does not exist. Diagnosis is based on the presence of a persistent fever along with the presence of various clinical features. The fever has to be present for at least five days (hence option "c" is false), and four of the following five criteria should be present:

1. *Bilateral conjunctival inflammation.* This is usually non-purulent and appears early in the illness and may therefore be mistaken for a viral conjunctivitis.
2. *Oropharyngeal changes.* These may include cracked, fissured and inflamed lips, an inflamed, non-purulent pharynx and strawberry tongue. These, in combination with fever, can easily be mistaken for a viral infection. A strawberry tongue is commonly associated with scarlet fever.
3. *A polymorphous rash.* The most non-specific of signs, the rash may be maculopapular (morbilliform), consist of discrete lesions (erythema multiforme) or be scarlatiniform (diffusely distributed numerous red papules), hence compounding the chances of a misdiagnosis.
4. *Cervical lymphadenopathy,* which may present in the form of a solitary lymph node. Can easily be confused with bacterial infection.
5. *Changes in the extremities.* These may include oedema and erythema. Late in the illness, desquamation of the fingers and toes tends to take place.

The above features tend not to appear together, making prompt diagnosis difficult. A high index of suspicion is required to make an accurate diagnosis, as the signs and symptoms unfold over the course of 5 to 10 days. Diagnostic accuracy is made more difficult by the presence of "incomplete Kawasaki disease", in which only two of the above features may be present with persistent fever. Although not diagnostic, acute phase reactants such as erythrocyte sedimentation rate (ESR) and C reactive protein (CRP) will be raised. White blood cell count is also likely to be raised, and they are worth measuring in the acute illness as subsequent measurements may help monitor disease activity.

Devastating complications: Prompt diagnosis of Kawasaki disease is important, as a missed, untreated episode carries a significant risk of serious consequences for the child. The major cause of morbidity and rarely, mortality is due to cardiovascular complications, specifically related to coronary artery disease that occurs as a result of the vasculitic process. Although coronary artery changes are seen in up to half of children with the illness, these will regress in the majority of cases. Some, however, will proceed to form aneurysms, which may stenose, thrombose or rupture. Worryingly, the dilatation of the coronary arteries may start within the first two weeks of developing fever. All children with a diagnosis of Kawasaki disease should have access to echocardiography in the acute phase of the illness, as this is a reliable method of detecting coronary artery aneurysms. It should be performed as soon as the diagnosis is suspected. Subsequent timings may be determined by the nature of the initial result. In uncomplicated cases, further echocardiograms should be performed at two weeks and then six to eight weeks from diagnosis. More frequent scans will be needed where complications are likely to develop (Newberger et al.). Other complications include myocarditis, pancarditis and rarely, heart failure. Long-term complications of the condition remain to be elucidated. A cohort of over 6000 patients with Kawasaki disease in childhood is being followed up in Japan (Nakamura et al., 2022). Some patients in the cohort are reaching their fourth decade. The hope is that they will help unravel the true impact of this intriguing condition on those who survive it into adulthood.

Effective treatment: A single infusion of intravenous immunoglobulin (IVIG), given at a dose of 2 g/kg, forms the mainstay of treatment of Kawasaki disease. It should be given between days 5 and 10 of the illness, with the onset of fever marking day 1 of the illness. It is effective in reducing fever within 36 hours of administration and reduces the risk of developing coronary artery aneurysms significantly. It can and should be administered after day 10 of the illness if the diagnosis was initially missed or if there is evidence of ongoing inflammation and fever. It is believed to work by having a generalized anti-inflammatory effect. Aspirin is used in conjunction with IVIG as an anti-inflammatory and antiplatelet agent. High doses are usually prescribed during the febrile phase, with a lower maintenance dose until a normal echocardiogram is seen at around six weeks. Aspirin does not appear to have a protective effect against the development of coronary artery disease. Other anti-inflammatory agents and treatment modalities that have been used in cases where fever persists despite IVIG include corticosteroids, plasmapheresis, cyclophosphamide, ciclosporin, ulinastatin (human trypsin inhibitor), abciximab (platelet glycoprotein IIb/IIIa receptor inhibitor) and infliximab (monoclonal antibodies against tumour necrosis factor α).

Learning Tip

Correctly identifying rare conditions is a hugely challenging and anxiety-provoking part of the practice of medicine. This can be made more challenging if the rare condition presents with a rare symptom. Managing patients presenting with a rare symptom offers quite a diagnostic conundrum. How does one determine whether there is underlying pathology to a bizarre symptom? One solution may be to consider the symptom in the context of the patient (Do they seem genuine, is there a history of bizarre presentations?), the nature of the symptom (Does it fit with any explainable biological system?) and any associated symptoms (Can they be connected to the rare symptom?). Some years ago, I saw a patient who kept seeing the face of his wife (who was with him) in everything that he saw. He seemed very genuine and had no other symptoms. It turned out that this rare symptom is known as palinopsia and in his case, was being caused by a brain tumour!

AKT PREPARATION

Options for questions 6–10:

a. McArdle syndrome
b. Wilson's disease
c. Von Gierke's disease
d. Wolman's disease
e. Glucose-6-phosphate dehydrogenase (G6PD) deficiency
f. Krabbe's disease
g. Menkes syndrome
h. Dubin–Johnson syndrome
i. Fanconi syndrome

Questions 6–10 are related to rare and eponymous disorders. Choose the most appropriate diagnosis from the list above for questions 6–10. Each option may be used once, more than once or not at all.

6. Low copper levels are associated with kinky, steel-like hair, osteoporosis, developmental retardation and seizures.

7. Enzyme deficiency leads to failure to dephosphorylate glucose-6-phosphate, resulting in lack of glucose production and possible hypoglycaemia.

8. Muscle phosphorylase deficiency leads to easy fatiguability during exercise.

9. Which of the following statements regarding congenital heart disease are true?

   a. Ebstein's anomaly has been linked with maternal lithium ingestion during pregnancy.
   b. A ventricular septal defect (VSD) is the commonest of the cyanotic congenital heart lesions.
   c. Coarctation of the aorta occurs more frequently in girls with Turner syndrome.
   d. Dextrocardia refers to an anatomically abnormal heart, more than half of which lies in the right side of the chest.
   e. Infants with tetralogy of Fallot are picked up at birth due to immediate cyanosis secondary to pulmonary stenosis.

10. Ten-year-old Joshua presents with Mum, who tells you that he has been complaining of left-sided chest pain for two weeks. On examination, you find an isolated, tender and mildly swollen second costochondral junction. What is the most likely diagnosis?

    a. Costochondritis
    b. Tietze's syndrome
    c. Slipping rib syndrome
    d. Texidor's twinge
    e. Pericarditis

BIBLIOGRAPHY

Buist NRM. Inborn errors of metabolism. In: Campbell AGM, McIntosh N. *Forfar & Arneil's Textbook of Pediatrics*. Churchill Livingstone; 1998. P. 1099–178.

Burns JC, Glode MP. Kawasaki syndrome. *Lancet* 2004; **364**:533–44.

Frank JE. Diagnosis and management of G6PD deficiency. *Am Fam Physician* 2005 Oct 1; **72**(7):1277–82.

Gardner-Medwin JM, Dolezalova P, Cummins C *et al*. Incidence of Henoch-Schönlein purpura, Kawasaki disease, and rare vasculitides in children of different ethnic origins. *Lancet* 2002; **360**(9341):1197–202.

Gordon JB, Kahn AM, Burns JC. When children with Kawasaki disease grow up: Myocardial and vascular complications in adulthood. *J Am Coll Cardiol* 2009; **54**(21):1911–20.

Harnden A, Alves B, Sheikh A. Rising incidence of Kawasaki disease in England: Analysis of hospital admission data. *BMJ* 2002; **324**(7351):1424–5.

Harnden A, Takahashi M, Burgner D. Kawasaki disease. *BMJ* 2009; **338**:b1514.

Houston AB. Cardiovascular disease. In: Campbell AGM, McIntosh N. *Forfar & Arneil's Textbook of Pediatrics*. Churchill Livingstone; 1998. P. 584–640.

Ives A, Daubeney PE, Balfour-Lynn IM. Recurrent chest pain in the well child. *Arch Dis Child* 2010 Aug; **95**(8):649–54.

McArdle B. Myopathy due to a defect in muscle glycogen breakdown. *Clin Sci* 1951 Feb; **10**(1):13–35.

Nakamura Y, Matsubara Y, Kosami K *et al.* Follow up of Kawasaki disease based on nationwide survey data in Japan: Mortality among those with a history of Kawasaki disease in Japan: Results of a 30-year follow up. *Pediatr Int* 2022; **64**(1):e15268.

Newburger JW, Takahashi M, Gerber MA *et al.* Diagnosis, treatment, and long-term management of Kawasaki disease: A statement for health professionals from the Committee on Rheumatic Fever, Endocarditis, and Kawasaki Disease, Council on Cardiovascular Disease in the Young, American Heart Association. *Pediatrics* 2004; **114**(6):1708–33.

Saguil A, Fargo M, Grogan S. Diagnosis and management of Kawasaki disease. *Am Fam Physician* 2015 Mar 15; **91**(6):365–71.

3

Case 3: Subclinical hypothyroidism

A 45-year-old female comes to see you for the third time in the month. She has had a difficult year with the loss of her job and dealing with the drug addiction of her 18-year-old son. Her main complaint, though, is feeling tired all the time. You organized some bloods on her first visit, which revealed a very minor iron deficiency, and prescribed her some iron replacement. This seems to have had very little effect on her symptoms. A colleague of yours prescribed her a short course of promethazine two weeks ago to help with her "stress-induced insomnia". This also, despite helping with the lack of sleep, did little to relieve her excessive tiredness. She enquires whether her tiredness may be linked with the abnormal thyroid blood test she noticed in the original results and would like to try a course of levothyroxine. You note that her thyroid-stimulating hormone (TSH) level was 6 mU/L with normal peripheral thyroid hormone levels. Further questioning does not reveal any other signs or symptoms of overt hypothyroidism.

Which of the following is the most appropriate next course of action?

a. Low-dose levothyroxine should be started to see if it will alleviate the symptoms of tiredness.
b. She should be reassured that her TSH, though slightly raised, is not the cause of her tiredness.
c. TSH levels should be repeated at an appropriate interval along with thyroid peroxidase (TPO) antibody levels.
d. Advise her that since her levels are only marginally abnormal, they can be rectified by adhering to a specific diet.
e. A lipid profile should be organized, and if abnormal, an appropriate dose of levothyroxine should be commenced.

DOI: 10.1201/9781003449737-4

ANSWER

c is correct

Subclinical hypothyroidism is considered, with a reasonable degree of expert agreement, to be early mild thyroid failure. However, much like other subclinical or preclinical entities in medicine, there is considerable debate on what implications it may have for the patient and when it should be considered an illness that needs treating. The upper limit of a normal TSH is debatable, and a different cut-off may be used by different laboratories, but it is usually set at around 4.5 mU/L (excluding pregnant women and the elderly). Some researchers have called for an even tighter definition of subclinical disease, suggesting an upper cut-off of 2.5 mU/L. This is based on population studies showing that 95% of the healthy population have TSH levels below this cut-off (Wartofsky, 2005). However, the implications for patient morbidity and benefits of treating at this level have not been well demonstrated; it may be associated with an increased risk of iatrogenic hyperthyroidism (Table 3.1).

In this case, it may be premature to start thyroid hormone replacement just yet. A TSH between 4.5 and 9 mU/L may be considered as representing mild subclinical hypothyroidism. Patients presenting with subclinical hypothyroidism with a TSH between 4 and 6 mU/L are more likely to revert to normal without intervention when compared with those with much higher TSH levels at diagnosis. TSH can be raised due to transient or physiological reasons (diurnal variation or recovery from illness), and therefore, a repeat blood test in the first instance is the most appropriate course of action. This, though, should not be a reason to dismiss the patient's symptoms either. Her TSH level is raised and therefore may be suggestive of early thyroid failure and hence responsible for her symptoms. The commonest cause of subclinical hypothyroidism is the presence of TPO antibodies, which indicate autoimmune thyroiditis (Hashimoto's disease). Therefore, a test for the antibodies should be performed along with the repeat blood for thyroid hormones. The presence of TPO antibodies, in the context of subclinical hypothyroidism, is associated with a higher risk of progression to overt hypothyroidism and would therefore justify more frequent monitoring of thyroid blood tests. There is no specific diet that helps thyroid disorders. Adequate iodine intake is important for optimal thyroid function, but a high iodine intake in subclinical hypothyroidism (in the presence of TPO antibodies) is associated with a greater risk of developing overt hypothyroidism.

Table 3.1   Aid to interpreting thyroid results

	TSH	FT4
Overt hypothyroidism	High	Low
Subclinical hypothyroidism	High	Normal
Secondary hypothyroidism	Normal or low	Low

> ### Learning Tip
>
> It is common in general practice to encounter scenarios where clinical presenta-
> tions don't quite neatly fit within the parameters of accepted guidelines. Variations
> of the above case for exam practice could include a pregnant woman, a patient
> with cardiovascular risk factors or an elderly patient. Familiarize yourself with the
> differences in management in these cases. The case can be made more challenging
> by the patient demanding medication in cases of mild subclinical hypothyroidism
> when immediate treatment may not be indicated. In such a case, a good grasp of
> the argument against treatment will be required to allow a seamless flow in the
> consultation.

Treatment in cases of subclinical hypothyroidism will be individualized depending on the extent and severity of the presenting symptoms, associated features such as cardiovascular risk and lipid profile, degree of thyroid dysfunction as evidenced by the blood results, and pregnancy status.

During pregnancy, the upper limit of TSH varies according to the trimester. Some authors have suggested a TSH above 2.5 mU/L in the first trimester and 3.5 mU/L in the second as suggestive of hypothyroidism, but a more sensible approach is to use local laboratory reference ranges, which reflect the local population. Some studies have shown a possible link between subclinical hypothyroidism and adverse effects on the pregnancy and cognitive impairment in the infant. As a result, some guidelines suggest checking for TPO antibodies in pregnant women with a TSH above 2.5 mU/L and treating if positive.

Another important determinant of whether treatment is indicated is the presence of cardiovascular risk factors. Some studies have suggested a possibility of increased risk of cardiovascular-related mortality with subclinical hypothyroidism, particularly in the young and middle-aged population. This should be discussed with patients who have the relevant risk factors to determine whether treatment is appropriate. Treatment may be more appropriate in this cohort when the TSH is above 10 mU/L due to the greater risk of progression to overt hypothyroidism and the greater likelihood that the patient will be symptomatic. If the TSH is below 10 mU/L and the patient is asymptomatic, a discussion with the patient with regard to the pros and cons of treatment will help reach a mutual decision as to how best to proceed.

Ageing itself can mimic symptoms of hypothyroidism (general slowing down, dry skin, intolerance of cold) but is not a "hypothyroid" state. Despite this, small rises in TSH are noted with increasing age. A US National Health and Nutritional Examination Survey (NHANES) III study found that the upper limit of normal in the above 80-year-old group could be as high as 7.9 mU/L. It is therefore reasonable to aim for a higher TSH when treating the elderly for subclinical hypothyroidism. A reasonable target would be a TSH of 4–7 mU/L, which should reduce the risk of the harms associated with iatrogenic hyperthyroidism.

AKT PREPARATION

Options for questions 11–15:

a. Start levothyroxine at 1.6 μg/kg
b. Start carbimazole
c. Start propylthiouracil
d. Increase dose of levothyroxine
e. Reduce dose of levothyroxine
f. Start beta-blocker
g. Add liothyronine
h. Start levothyroxine at 25 μg a day
i. None of the above

Questions 11–15 refer to the management of thyroid disease. From the list, choose the most appropriate (first-line) management plan for each scenario. Each option may be used once, more than once or not at all.

Serum-free T4 reference range: 11.2–20.2 pmol/L

11. A 65-year-old male with a history of ischaemic heart disease has the following results: TSH 15 mU/L, serum-free T4 level 4.6 pmol/L.

12. A 37-year-old female has the following results: TSH <0.01 mU/L, serum T4 level 12.8. Her T3 level is normal.

13. A 30-year-old female with no previous medical history has the following results: TSH 18 mU/L, serum T4 level 4.5 pmol/L.

14. Subclinical hyperthyroidism is defined by a low TSH but normal T4 and triiodothyronine (T3) levels. Which of the following is false?

    a. Serum TSH levels tend to be lower in black people when compared with white people.
    b. Lower serum TSH concentrations can be seen in healthy smokers.
    c. Toxic multinodular goitre is the commonest cause of subclinical hyperthyroidism in young people.
    d. A low serum TSH may be seen at the end of the first trimester due to stimulation of the thyroid by placental human chorionic gonadotrophin (hCG).
    e. Low levels of TSH can be seen with glucocorticoid treatment.

15. Which of the following features is not part of the Burch–Wartofsky Point Scale (BWPS) for the diagnosis of thyrotoxicosis?

a. Temperature °F (°C) >99 (37.2)
b. Delirium
c. Unexplained jaundice
d. Heart rate >90
e. T4 40 pmol/L

BIBLIOGRAPHY

Alexander EK, Marqusee E, Lawrence J et al. Timing and magnitude of increases in levothyroxine requirements during pregnancy in women with hypothyroidism. *N Engl J Med* 2004; **351**:241–9.

Alexander EK, Pearce E, Brent G et al. Guidelines of the American Thyroid Association for the diagnosis and management of thyroid disease during pregnancy and the postpartum. *Thyroid* 2017; **27**:315–89.

Cooper DS, Biondi B. Subclinical thyroid disease. *Lancet* 2012 Mar 24; **379**(9821):1142–54.

Deshauer S, Wyne A. Subclinical hypothyroidism in pregnancy. *CMAJ* 2017; **189**:E941.

Diez JJ, Iglesias P, Burman K D. Spontaneous normalization of thyrotropin concentrations in patients with subclinical hypothyroidism. *J Clin Endocrinol Metab* 2005 Jul; **90**(7):4124–7.

Fatourechi V. Subclinical hypothyroidism: An update for primary care physicians. *Mayo Clin Proc* 2009 Jan; **84**(1):65–71.

Hollowell JG, Staehling NW, Flanders WD, et al. Serum TSH, T_4, and thyroid antibodies in the United States population (1988 to 1994): National Health and Nutrition Examination Survey (NHANES III) *J Clin Endocrinol Metab* 2002; **87**:489–99.

Leng O, Razvi S. Hypothyroidism in the older population. *Thyroid Res* 2019; **12**:2.

Li Y, Teng D, Shan Z et al. Antithyroperoxidase and Antithyroglobulin antibodies in a five-year follow-up survey of populations with different iodine intakes. *J Clin Endocrinol Metab* 2008; **93**:1751–7.

Vaidya B, Pearce SHS. Management of hypothyroidism in adults. *BMJ* 2008; **337**:a801.

Waise A, Price HC. The upper limit of the reference range for thyroid-stimulating hormone should not be confused with a cut-off to define subclinical hypothyroidism. *Ann Clin Biochem* 2009 Mar; **46**(Pt 2):93–8.

Wartofsky L, Dickey RA. The evidence for a narrower thyrotropin reference range is compelling. *J Clin Endocrinol Metab* 2005 Sep; **90**(9):5483–8.

Wilber JF, Utiger RD. The effect of glucocorticoids on thyrotropin secretion. *J Clin Invest* 1969 Nov; **48**(11):2096–103.

4

Case 4: Hyperemesis gravidarum

A 22-year-old woman sees you in surgery for pregnancy counselling. She has a two-year-old healthy son. During the first trimester of her pregnancy with him, she suffered from severe vomiting for the first 10 weeks. At first, it was managed with oral antiemetics and fluid therapy at home. Eventually, her situation deteriorated to a point where hospital admission became necessary. She recalls that she was losing an alarming amount of weight in hospital due to the vomiting, and it was eventually decided to start her on steroids. This eventually managed to bring the situation under control. However, she remembers being told that the steroids increased the risk of her child developing cleft palate. At the time, she had vowed not to get pregnant again, but is now wondering if that was a sensible decision. She is keen for another child and wanted your opinion regarding this. She is particularly interested in knowing if she can take any measures to prevent a repeat of the problems of the last pregnancy.

Which of the following statements is false?

a. Her risk of developing hyperemesis gravidarum (HG) in the second pregnancy is higher than the background risk of 1/200 pregnancies.
b. Multiple pregnancy is associated with a higher risk of developing HG.
c. HG is associated with a transient hypothyroidism, thought to be due to the similarities in molecular structure of thyroid-stimulating hormone (TSH) and human chorionic gonadotrophin (hCG).
d. Ginger has been shown to be beneficial in reducing nausea and vomiting in early pregnancy.
e. Acupuncture may be safely used as an option in the treatment of vomiting in pregnancy.

DOI: 10.1201/9781003449737-5

ANSWER

c is false

Nausea and vomiting in the early stages of pregnancy are extremely common, affecting more than half of pregnancies. Hyperemesis gravidarum represents the most extreme form of this condition. Vomiting in HG is persistent, causing more than 5% weight loss and accompanied with ketosis. Electrolyte imbalances are also commonly seen. These include low levels of magnesium, phosphate and potassium. Urea and creatinine levels may be raised, and liver function tests may be grossly abnormal. Jaundice, however, is very uncommon. HG is thankfully uncommon, affecting about 0.5–1% of pregnancies. Unfortunately, due to a previous episode, the risk may be as high as 15% in our patient. This is a distressing condition, usually leaving the pregnant woman exhausted and away from family and work. As was the case in her first pregnancy, it can be quite difficult to treat, requiring treatments that may potentially harm the growing fetus. As discussed in the previous case, HG is associated with a transient hyperthyroidism due to thyroid stimulation by hCG, which is a weak TSH agonist. This hyperthyroidism does not need treating and will normally resolve by the 18th week of the pregnancy. Higher levels of hCG, such as are found in multiple and molar pregnancy, are also associated with HG. The severity of symptoms seems to correlate with higher levels of hCG. Conditions such as hydatiform mole and choriocarcinoma, which are associated with very high levels of hCG, can precipitate gestational thyrotoxicosis (Hershman, 1999).

This patient will naturally be concerned about her risk of getting HG again in this pregnancy. Although the risk of developing HG is greater, being mentally prepared may improve her chances of being able to deal with it. Our job is to maximize the chances of this. Strategies that may help in improving her ability to cope with HG may include:

- The availability of good family support may reduce the risk of developing HG and also reduce its intensity.
- Access to psychosocial support should be discussed. Show understanding of the fact that HG can cause considerable physical and psychological distress.
- Foods that trigger symptoms of nausea and vomiting should be avoided.
- If the patient is on iron supplements, it should be considered whether it is possible to stop them. This has been shown to reduce the symptoms of nausea and vomiting early in pregnancy Although not known to specifically help against developing HG, folic acid supplements should be encouraged pre-fertilization.
- *Helicobacter pylori* has also been implicated in the development of HG. One may screen for this and treat if indicated.
- A thyroid function test may be performed to determine the pre-conceptual thyroid status.
- One study has shown that pre-emptive treatment with antiemetics, prior to conception, may reduce the risk of developing troublesome symptoms in women who had severe symptoms in a previous pregnancy (Koren, 2004).

Pharmacologically, antihistamines are usually the first-line antiemetics used in the treatment of nausea, vomiting and HG. There is good evidence for them being safe in pregnancy. Promethazine and prochlorperazine are commonly used. Metoclopramide, a dopamine antagonist, is also an effective choice but is recommended as a second-line choice due to the risk of extrapyramidal side effects. The 5HT3 receptor antagonist ondansetron, commonly prescribed for post-operative and chemotherapy-related nausea and vomiting, has been shown to be of use in severe cases of HG. Studies have also shown diazepam to be effective in treating nausea in pregnancy, but use remains limited due to concerns regarding its addictive potential. The use of steroids is slightly controversial, though they have been shown to be effective in treating intractable hyperemesis. There are concerns regarding their teratogenic potential, with some studies suggesting a three-fold increase in the risk of developing cleft palate. Their use is limited to secondary care. Pyridoxine (Vitamin B6) has been shown to be beneficial for pregnancy-induced nausea. One study showed that when taken at 30 mg once daily, it caused a significant reduction in nausea when compared with placebo. Although it reduced vomiting also, the difference was not significant. Pyridoxine is not recommended for use in the National Institute for Health and Care Excellence (NICE) accredited Royal College of Obstetricians and Gynaecologists (RCOG) guidelines. It is, however, recommended by both the American and Canadian guidelines at a dose of up to 40 mg daily to help prevent pregnancy-induced nausea. It should be used with an antihistamine and started as soon as the early symptoms develop to prevent their worsening. In the UK, it is available in combination with the selective H_1 receptor antihistamine doxylamine. Ginger has also been shown to be a useful option in HG. A double-blind randomized controlled trial (RCT) of 30 women found that 1 g of powdered root of ginger (taken as 250 mg four times a day) was better than placebo at reducing symptoms of HG. It does not appear to have any significant side effects (Fischer-Rasmussen, 1991).

Acupuncture and acupressure are non-pharmacological means by which women may seek to overcome nausea and vomiting in pregnancy. They certainly seem to be safe, a fact reflected in the RCOG guidelines, which recommend acupressure along with ginger and antihistamines as the three treatment options for this condition (hypnosis, though, is not recommended). A study by Neri and colleagues compared acupuncture and acupressure versus metoclopramide and vitamin B12 supplementation in 88 women suffering from HG. The effect of pharmacotherapy was immediate, whereas the acupuncture group benefitted most towards the end of the two-week period. Both methods were effective in reducing vomiting. Acupuncture seemed to have a more favourable effect on daily functioning. Acupressure was applied for six to eight hours a day, which may represent a limitation to its use. It can certainly be recommended to patients as an alternative to pharmacotherapy if the symptoms are not severe.

A recent breakthrough study (Fejzo et al., 2023) has shed new light on the potential underlying cause of HG. GDF15, a hormone produced by the fetus, acts on the maternal brainstem to trigger nausea, vomiting and in severe cases, HG. GDF15 is made by other tissues of the body outside pregnancy. It appears that low pre-pregnancy exposure to GDF15 renders the mother more sensitive to the sudden increase in circulating GDF15 that is produced by the fetus. This, in turn, triggers the symptoms of HG. A rare genetic variant was identified that resulted in low circulating levels of GDF15, predisposing the possessors of this variant to a higher risk of developing HG. Interestingly, beta-thalassaemia trait is associated with chronically high levels of GDF15 and therefore acts as a protective factor against the development of HG. These findings raise the hope of developing novel treatment options for patients suffering from this debilitating condition.

> **Learning Tip**
>
> Providing reassurance to our patients is a key part of our job. Reassurance may be affective or cognitive. Affective reassurance refers to the process of building rapport with the patient and demonstrating empathy. This gives patients the sense that they are being cared for and their fears and worries are understood and respected. Cognitive reassurance involves health education by explaining the nature of the medical problem being discussed and clear management plans. This empowers the patient and encourages self-management of problems, where possible. A successful consultation will employ both forms of reassurance, hence maximizing positive outcomes for the patient.

AKT PREPARATION

Options for questions 16–20:

a. Hyperemesis gravidarum
b. Obstetric cholestasis
c. Pre-eclampsia
d. Budd–Chiari syndrome
e. HELLP syndrome
f. Wilson's disease
g. Acute fatty liver of pregnancy
h. Drug-induced hepatotoxicity
i. None of the above

Questions 16–20 relate to pregnant women presenting with liver disorders in pregnancy. Pick the most suitable diagnosis suggested by the combination of signs, symptoms and investigations. Each answer may be used once, more than once or not at all.

16. A 34-week pregnant woman presents with itching of her palms and soles. There is no visible rash. A blood test reveals a bile acid concentration of 34 µmol/L (normal <10 µmol/L).

17. A 16-week pregnant woman presents with generalized fatigue, which started before conception. She reports troublesome pruritis for the last three months. Blood tests show elevated aminotransferases and alkaline phosphatase and the presence of anti-mitochondrial antibodies (AMA).

18. A 40-year-old woman presents in the third trimester of her pregnancy with right upper quadrant and epigastric pain. Her blood pressure is recorded at 120/80 mmHg, and she has 3+ proteinuria on urine dip measurement. Bloods reveal a reduced haemoglobin level, elevated aspartate aminotransferase at 90 IU/L, raised lactate dehydrogenase at 800 IU/L and low platelet levels at 76 × 10⁹/L.

19. Which of the following statements regarding liver disease in pregnancy are true?

   a. If vomiting persists beyond the 18th gestational week, a gastroscopy should be considered to rule out a mechanical obstruction.
   b. The presence of oedema of the hands and feet is necessary for the diagnosis of pre-eclampsia.
   c. The Tennessee system and the Mississippi system are classification systems used in HELLP syndrome.
   d. The incidence of Budd–Chiari syndrome is increased in pregnancy.
   e. The Swansea diagnostic criteria are used in the diagnosis of intrahepatic cholestasis of pregnancy.

20. Pick the one true statement from the options below.

   a. If needed, hepatitis B vaccine (HBV) can be given safely in pregnancy.
   b. Breastfeeding is the most common mode of transmission of HBV worldwide.
   c. HBV viral load appears to have no effect on the risk of vertical transmission.
   d. Caesarean section reduces the risk of vertical transmission of HBV.
   e. The risk of vertical transmission of hepatitis C virus (HCV) is high in HIV-negative mothers.

BIBLIOGRAPHY

Crosignani A, Battezzati PM, Invernizzi P et al. Clinical features and management of primary biliary cirrhosis. World J Gastroenterol 2008; 14(21):3313–27.

Fejzo M, Rocha N, Cimino I et al. GDF15 linked to maternal risk of nausea and vomiting during pregnancy. Nature 2023; 625(7996):760–7.

Fischer-Rasmussen W, Kjaer SK, Dahl C, Asping U. Ginger treatment of hyperemesis gravidarum. Eur J Obstet Gynecol Reprod Biol Jan 1991; 4(38):19–24.

Gadsby R, Barnie-Adshead T. Severe nausea and vomiting of pregnancy: Should it be treated with appropriate pharmacotherapy? Obstet Gynaecol 2011; 13:107–11.

Girling J, Knight CL, Chappell L; on behalf of the Royal College of Obstetricians and Gynaecologists. Intrahepatic cholestasis of pregnancy. BJOG 2022; 129(13):e95–e114.

Hershman JM. Human chorionic gonadotropin and the thyroid: Hyperemesis gravidarum and trophoblastic tumors. Thyroid 1999 Jul; 9(7):653–7.

Jeanneret M, Dawlatly B. Severe hyperemesis on a background of gatsroparesis. J Obs Gynecol July 2009; 29(5):437–8.

Joshi D, James A, Quaglia A, Westbrook RH, Heneghan MA. Liver disease in pregnancy. *Lancet* Feb 2010; **375**:594–605.

Kaplan MM, Gershwin ME. Primary biliary cirrhoisis. *N Engl J Med* 2005; **353**:1261–73.

Koren G, Maltepe C. Pre-emptive therapy for severe nausea and vomiting of pregnancy and hyperemesis gravidarum. *J Obstet Gynaecol* 2004 Aug; **24**(5):530–3.

Neri I, Allais G, Schiapparelli P, Blasi I, Benedetto C, Facchinetti F. Acupuncture versus pharmacological approach to reduce Hyperemesis gravidarum discomfort. *Minerva Ginecol* Aug 2005; **57**(4):471–5.

Pincus T, Holt N, Vogel S *et al.* Cognitive and affective reassurance and patient outcomes in primary care: A systematic review. *Pain* 2013; **154**(11):2407–16.

RCOG. *The Management of Nausea and Vomiting of Pregnancy and Hyperemesis Gravidarum*. Green-Top Guideline No. 69. RCOG; June 2016.

Tamay AG, Kuscu NK. Hyperemesis gravidarum: Current aspects. *J Obs Gynecol* 2011 Nov; **31**:708–12.

Vutyavanich T, Wongtrangan S, Ruangsri R. Pyridoxine for nausea and vomiting of pregnancy: A randomized, double-blind, placebo-controlled trial. *Am J Obstet Gynecol* 1995 Sep; **173**:881–4.

Case 5: Tinnitus

5

A 56-year-old male, who works as a construction worker, presents with a six-month history of tinnitus. He describes it as a continuous humming or hissing sound, which seems to originate from the centre of his head. He does not recall the exact moment it started, but it seems to have become more noticeable with the passage of time. He describes it being worse when he is trying to sleep at night. He has not noticed any issues with his hearing. He previously completed a tinnitus functional index (TFI) and got a score of 80 (which correlates with the tinnitus being a moderate problem). He finds that his sleep is interrupted as a result, which is affecting his ability to work effectively the next day. He has a past medical history of polymyalgia rheumatica and is currently on a reducing dose of prednisolone. He would like to know what can be done to help alleviate his symptoms.

Which of the following statements is/are true?

a. The homogeneity of tinnitus experience and presentation lends it well to treatment research.
b. In the absence of an underlying cause, betahistine is recommended as first-line treatment for tinnitus.
c. Prednisolone has been implicated as a potential ototoxic drug that may cause tinnitus.
d. There is no benefit in carrying out an audiological assessment, as the patient does not report any hearing loss.
e. The patient should be reassured that the prevalence of tinnitus reduces with age, and thus, his symptoms are likely to self-resolve.

ANSWER

c is true

Tinnitus can be defined as the perception of a sound in the absence of an external auditory stimulus (Ralli, 2017). The sound perceived may be described in a variety of ways by the patient and can include a hissing, buzzing or ringing or even a voice or music (auditory or musical imagery tinnitus). The sound can be heard in either ear, in the middle of the head or even the outside of the head, or in a difficult-to-localize place. The tinnitus may be intermittent, continuous and/or pulsatile. All these features contribute to the heterogeneity of tinnitus, lending it poorly to objective clinical research. This is likely a major cause of the paucity of understanding of the condition and the lack of evidence-based treatments available.

Tinnitus prevalence seems to increase up to the age of 70; whether the prevalence increases or decreases beyond 70 is unclear, as studies have shown conflicting evidence. However, the patient can be reassured that in a significant number of people, the tinnitus can spontaneously disappear or at least diminish in its severity. It seems that one of the mechanisms for explaining tinnitus is the brain becoming more sensitive to background noise in the presence of sensory deprivation during high-frequency hearing loss. This may explain why tinnitus is at its most annoying when things are quiet or when trying to sleep in the stillness of the night. The gradual habituation of the brain to the sensory deprivation may explain the eventual recovery from tinnitus as the brain "stops scanning" for a background signal.

Hearing loss is the commonest cause of tinnitus and is therefore more likely to be seen in patients who are exposed to high levels of noise either at work or during recreation. Construction or manufacturing workers working with tools, musicians or those in the armed forces may be considered as being at high risk of occupational noise exposure. Even though our patient does not report any hearing loss, it would be prudent to carry out an objective audiological assessment. Moreover, corticosteroids, which our case patient has been using, have been linked with ototoxicity and hence the development of tinnitus.

The National Institute of Health and Care Excellence (NICE) recommends the use of scoring scales such as the TFI where appropriate. The TFI scores patients on various aspects of the tinnitus, such as the loudness, subjective sense of control over the tinnitus and its effect on one's ability to sleep, relax, concentrate and generally enjoy life. The final score is divided into five categories, with categories 4 and 5 correlating with severe tinnitus.

Betahistine is not recommended for the treatment of isolated tinnitus due to the lack of evidence for its efficacy. It has a role to play if the tinnitus is part of Ménière's disease, which is discussed later.

> **Learning Tip**
>
> Tinnitus can make an interesting Simulated Consultation Assessment (SCA) preparation case. In many cases, there may not be an underlying cause of the tinnitus. However, there are many interesting risk factors and conditions that are associated with tinnitus. The presenting case can be as above, where there is no treatable cause for the tinnitus, or it can be a symptom of another condition.
>
> A few of these conditions and their peculiarities in terms of management are discussed below. This should give the trainee a more broad understanding of tinnitus and the pitfalls to look out for, and serve as a base for managing the medical complexity that may present with tinnitus.

SCA BONUS CASE 1: VESTIBULAR SCHWANNOMA

A 66-year-old male presents with unilateral tinnitus and profound hearing loss in the same ear, which has been gradually progressing over the last six months.

More commonly known as an acoustic neuroma, a vestibular schwannoma is a benign tumour arising from the Schwann cells of the vestibulocochlear nerve (8th cranial nerve). It most commonly presents with unilateral hearing loss, with tinnitus being the second most common presenting symptom. Other symptoms include dizziness, ataxia and a loss of balance. As the tumour grows, it can press on the nearby trigeminal and facial nerves, causing numbness in the face and paralysis. Any patient presenting with unilateral hearing loss and tinnitus should have a magnetic resonance imaging (MRI) scan done. Management is carried out by specialist teams and can involve microsurgery, radiosurgery or a watch-and-wait approach, depending on the size of the tumour and its rate of growth in relation to the age of the patient.

SCA BONUS CASE 2: MÉNIÈRE'S DISEASE

A 50-year-old woman presents with a third episode in six months of intense vertigo, tinnitus, loss of hearing and a pressure-like sensation in her right ear. Her second "attack" led to a three-day admission to hospital, where a host of cardiac and neurological investigations failed to demonstrate a cause for her symptoms.

A 50 year old presenting with vertigo, tinnitus, loss of hearing and a sensation of fullness in the ear is likely to have Ménière's disease. The symptoms may not occur in that order, and the vertigo in particular can be quite sudden and disabling. Named after the French physician Prosper Ménière, the symptoms of the condition are thought to be caused by the abnormal build-up of endolymphatic fluid in the vestibular and cochlear compartments of the inner ear. The exact aetiology and pathophysiology of the condition, however, remain elusive, and it continues to be a diagnosis of exclusion once other causes of hearing loss, dizziness and tinnitus have been ruled out. It is only after multiple presentations of acute vertigo, vomiting and tinnitus (often confused with gastroenteritis on first presentation) and subsequent normal investigations that the diagnosis is usually made. Evidence for the treatment of Ménière's disease remains scant, but treatment options include betahistine, thiazide diuretics, intratympanic gentamicin or steroid injections, endolymphatic sac surgery and pressure pulse therapy. This involves controlled micro-pressure pulses, delivered into the inner ear via a ventilation tube in the tympanic membrane by an externally placed device. Patients are generally advised to adhere to a low salt diet and reduce caffeine and alcohol intake, although the evidence for the efficacy of such advice is poor.

OTHER CAUSES

Ultimately, tinnitus can be associated with a whole host of other conditions, the treatment of which, if available, is likely to lead to resolution of the tinnitus. Age-related hearing loss is amongst the commonest causes of tinnitus and can be rectified by offering the patient a hearing amplification device. There is no benefit in offering an amplification device for tinnitus in the absence of any objective hearing loss. Tinnitus can be experienced with any otological infection such as otitis media, labyrinthitis and vestibular neuritis. Impacted earwax can also cause tinnitus and is a common problem seen in primary care. Tinnitus can be associated with head injury and can unfortunately persist beyond recovery from the initial insult. Hypertension has long been recognized as being associated with tinnitus, caused perhaps by microvascular destruction of the inner ear or increased perception of the noise of the blood vessels in the vicinity of the inner ear. However, antihypertensive drugs such as diuretics, beta-blockers, angiotensin-converting enzyme inhibitors (ACE-i), angiotensin II receptor blockers (ARBs) and calcium channel blockers have been implicated as possible ototoxic medications. Any form of stress, anxiety and depression is also linked with tinnitus, with existing tinnitus often getting worse with any new emotional trauma. It is important to explore this in all patients presenting with tinnitus. Other related conditions (non-exhaustive) include temporomandibular joint disorder, thyroid disease, migraine, epilepsy and multiple sclerosis.

RED FLAGS

Red flags in the case of tinnitus do not necessarily represent acute and urgent pathology indicative of an emergency but rather, warrant further investigations through specialist referral:

- *Tinnitus is audible to an observer.* This rare phenomenon is known as objective tinnitus, and the sound can be heard by the examiner by either placing a stethoscope near the ear or being in very close vicinity to it. This may represent an arteriovenous malformation, stenosis in the carotid or vertebral artery, or even a vascular tumour. Although rare, it should not be ignored and warrants further investigations.
- *Pulsatile tinnitus.* Although this may be caused by stress or acute ear inflammatory conditions, a vascular cause will need to be ruled out if the pulsatile tinnitus

(particularly if synchronous with the heartbeat) cannot be attributed to benign or self-limiting causes. An asynchronous pulsatile tinnitus may be caused by spasms in the middle ear or palatal muscles.

- *Tinnitus with hearing loss.* NICE guidelines suggest specialist referral; and for the patient to be seen within 24 hours if hearing loss has developed suddenly (over a period of 3 days or less) in the past 30 days.
- *Acute tinnitus after head injury* warrants urgent imaging.
- *Tinnitus with acute neurological signs and symptoms or uncontrolled vestibular symptoms.* Refer immediately.
- *Tinnitus as part of a psychological presentation* with high risk of suicide requires urgent referral to mental health services.

MANAGEMENT

As should be fairly clear by now, the causes of tinnitus are multitudinous, and the primary management revolves around treating the underlying cause. The final part of this case will focus on the management of the tinnitus when there is no reversible cause or where the tinnitus has persisted despite treating the original underlying cause.

The most important aspect of the management of tinnitus is reassurance. Patients should be provided with information leaflets, which are likely to help them to come to terms with their symptoms. Lifestyle advice around reducing stress is also likely to help. Most importantly, the symptom should not be belittled or its effect on the patient played down.

Although drugs do not cure tinnitus, they can help in alleviating the severity of the symptoms of tinnitus when it is not due to a specific or treatable cause. The poor availability of other treatment modalities discussed below may mean that drugs end up being the first port of call in the management of tinnitus. Centrally acting drugs such as amitriptyline, acamprosate and gabapentin have been shown to improve tinnitus severity. The anti-inflammatory effect of an intratympanic injection of dexamethasone has also been associated with a reduction in the severity of tinnitus and can be carried out under specialist supervision. If sleep is significantly affected, then a short-term sedative may be appropriate but is not an appropriate long-term strategy. Melatonin has shown some potential in patients with tinnitus and may have a role to play in tinnitus associated with sleep disruption. Although no evidence exists for the treatment of tinnitus by complementary medicine, it may offer some help by inducing relaxation in patients and therefore may be tried.

Other treatment options include:

- Cognitive behavioural therapy.
- Sound therapy covers a wide array of technologies, from recorded sounds to be played in the background to wearable sound generators that aim to mask the tinnitus. There are various commercially produced devices, which ideally should be used alongside education and psychological therapies.
- Brain stimulation remains an area of research for the treatment of tinnitus.

- Surgery for tinnitus remains a niche approach, but targeting neurovascular compressions around the auditory nerve may represent a target for surgical interventions.

AKT PREPARATION

Options for questions 21–25:

a. Acute glaucoma
b. Scleritis
c. Anterior uveitis
d. Viral conjunctivitis
e. Chemosis
f. Endophthalmitis
g. Periorbital cellulitis
h. Episcleritis
i. Herpes zoster ophthalmicus

Questions 21–25 relate to ophthalmological problems. For each question, pick the most likely diagnosis from the list above. Each answer may be used once, more than once or not at all.

21. One week after cataract surgery, a 64-year-old man presents with a painful red eye, reduced vision and sensitivity to light. A hypopyon is visible, and an intraocular culture is positive for bacteria.

22. A 70-year-old woman presents one week after starting amitriptyline for diabetes-induced neuropathy. She presents with an acutely painful red eye, nausea and vomiting, headache and reduced visual acuity.

23. An 18-year-old boy with known hay fever presents during pollen season with a visible jelly-like swelling on the eyeball. He had been cutting grass in his garden and developed itchiness in the eye prior to the swelling appearing. His vision is unaffected, but the eye is red and itchy.

24. Which of the following statements regarding eczema herpeticum are false?

    a. Most cases of eczema herpeticum are caused by herpes zoster virus.
    b. Recurrent episodes of eczema herpeticum are uncommon.
    c. All children should be treated with intravenous antiviral treatment.
    d. Antibiotic treatment is usually required to treat bacterial superinfection.
    e. Untreated, eczema herpeticum is potentially fatal.

25. Which of the following is/are complications of a cholesteatoma?

    a. Facial palsy
    b. Hearing loss
    c. Meningitis
    d. Labyrinthine fistula
    e. Vertigo

BIBLIOGRAPHY

Baguley D, McFerran D, Hall D. Tinnitus. *Lancet* 2013; **382**:1600–7.

Chang P, Kim S. Cholesteatoma – Diagnosing the unsafe ear. *Aust Fam Physician* 2008; **37**(8):631–8.

Chen J, Chen Y, Zeng B *et al*. Efficacy of pharmacologic treatment in tinnitus patients without specific or treatable origin: A network meta-analysis of randomised controlled trials. *EClinicalMedicine* 2021 Aug 13; **39**:101080.

David TJ, Longson M. Herpes simplex infections in atopic eczema. *Arch Dis Child* 1985 April; **60**(4):338–43.

Durand ML. Endophthalmitis. *Clin Microbiol Infect* 2013 Mar; **19**(3):227–34.

Figueiredo RR, Azevedo AA, Penido NDO. Positive association between tinnitus and arterial hypertension. *Front Neurol* 2016; **7**:171.

Foley RW, Shirazi S, Maweni RM *et al*. Signs and symptoms of acoustic neuroma at initial presentation: An exploratory analysis. *Cureus* 2017 Nov; **9**(11):e184.

Hannan SA, Sami F, Wareing MJ. Tinnitus. *BMJ* 2005 Jan 29; **330**(7485):237.

House JW, Brackmann DE. Tinnitus: Surgical treatment. *Ciba Found Symp* 1981; **85**:204–16.

Liddle BJ. Herpes simplex infections in atopic eczema. *Arch Dis Child* 1990 Mar; **65**(3):333.

Luca PD, Cassandro C, Ralli M *et al*. Dietary restriction for the treatment of Ménière's disease. *Transl Med UniSa* 2020 May; **22**:5–9.

Merrick L, Youssef D, Tanner M, Peiris AN. Does melatonin have therapeutic use in tinnitus? *South Med J* 2014 Jun;**107**(6):362–6.

Pohl H, Tarnutzer AA. Acute angle-closure glaucoma. *N Engl J Med* 2018 Mar 8; **378**(10):e14.

Ralli M, Balla MP, Greco A *et al*. Work-related noise exposure in a cohort of patients with chronic tinnitus: Analysis of demographic and audiological characteristics. *Int J Environ Res Public Health* 2017 Sep; **14**(9):1035.

Tinnitus: Assessment and Management. NICE Guideline NG155. 2020. https://www.nice.org.uk/guidance/ng155/chapter/Recommendations#management-of-tinnitus

van Esch BF, van der Zaag-Loonen H, Bruintjes T *et al*. Interventions for Ménière's disease: An umbrella systematic review. *BMJ Evid-Based Med* 2022; **27**:235–45.

6

Case 6: Febrile seizures

You see a 15-month-old child in clinic with a 24-hour history of fever, runny nose and tugging at the right ear. The child appears well on examination and is afebrile. You note that the right tympanic membrane is bulging with an inflamed appearance. You make a diagnosis of otitis media and send Mum home with a prescription of amoxicillin. Two days later, Mum, who is an orthopaedic nurse, returns with discharge papers from the paediatric ward. Later at night after you saw him, the child developed a very high tempera-ture of 39 degrees. As he lay in his cot, he suddenly started jerking. Mum says he appeared to go very stiff and became unresponsive with his eyes rolled upwards. Thinking that he was dying, Mum dialled for the ambulance. By the time the ambulance crew arrived, the jerking had settled. He, however, remained semi-conscious, and it was not until an hour later in the emergency department that he was completely back to normal. The paediatric discharge notes inform you that a lumbar puncture was performed. It, along with blood results, was normal. The final diagnosis was that of a simple febrile seizure (FS). Mum would like the child to be referred for an electroencephalogram (EEG). She also enquires about prophylactic diazepam to stop seizures from occurring in the future.

Which of the following statements is/are true?

a. A lumbar puncture is always indicated when a child presents with a FS.
b. It is good practice to perform blood tests to get an idea regarding the severity of the infection.
c. An EEG should have been carried out during the admission, as it is a most sensitive test when carried out within 24 hours of the seizure.
d. Long-term outcome after a febrile seizure is excellent in terms of intellectual capa-bility and behaviour.
e. There is strong and convincing evidence that febrile seizures cause damage to the hippocampus, resulting in an increased risk of developing temporal lobe epilepsy (TLE).

ANSWER

d is true

Febrile seizures are a commonly encountered paediatric problem, occurring in 2% to 5% of all children. There are slight variations in how a FS may be defined; however, it is commonly described as a seizure associated with fever in the absence of underlying intracranial infection or any other recognized cause of seizure activity such as trauma, epilepsy or electrolyte imbalance. They are more common in children between the ages of six months and three years, with a peak incidence at the age of 18 months. Onset after the age of six is uncommon. A fever of greater than 38 °C is usually quoted as being required to make the diagnosis of a FS. Despite this, the fever may not be the cause of the FS. This is backed by studies showing that the use of antipyretics is not effective in preventing the recurrence of febrile seizures. A randomized double-blind, placebo-controlled trial performed by Stuijvenberg and colleagues randomized 230 children between the ages of one and four to receive either ibuprofen or placebo regularly during a febrile episode until adequate temperature control had been achieved. These children had had a febrile seizure in the past and were deemed at high risk of having a recurrence. Analysis at the end of the study did not show any difference in the risk of recurrent FSs. Other studies have yielded similar results with paracetamol. It is possible that endogenous proteins such as interleukin 1, released during a pyretic episode, increase neuronal excitability and lower the seizure threshold, thus linking the fever with the seizure. The exact mechanism, however, remains elusive.

The strongest risk factor for having a FS is a history of FSs in a first-degree relative. For most children, this will be a solitary event; however, a FS will recur in approximately a third of children. They are at the highest risk within the first year of the initial event. FSs may be classified as follows:

- *Simple.* Simple seizures, which make up the large majority of FSs, are short in duration (lasting less than 10 minutes), have generalized tonic–clonic seizure activity, resolve spontaneously and do not recur within 24 hours.
- *Complex.* Seizures are classified as complex if they last for longer than 15 minutes, have focal seizure activity or reoccur within 24 hours. Febrile status epilepticus is a form of complex FS in which the seizure lasts for greater than 30 minutes.

The differentiation is important, as a complex FS is associated with an increased risk of developing epilepsy when compared with a simple FS (if all three features are present, the risk of developing epilepsy is approximately 50%). Other factors increasing the risk of developing epilepsy include a family history of epilepsy and neurological abnormalities. Interestingly, fever duration of less than one hour prior to seizure onset is also associated with an increased risk of developing epilepsy later in life. In contrast, a simple FS with none of the above factors is associated with a 2.4% risk of developing epilepsy (a modest rise above the 1.4% risk for the background population). Parents should be reassured that long-term prognosis in terms of intellect, academic achievement, memory and behaviour is good.

The first step in the management is to confirm the diagnosis. As is the case in the scenario above, it is not uncommon for seizure activity to have terminated by the time the child reaches the emergency department. As with all cases, a good history is vital. Alternative diagnoses, including rigors, syncope, reflex anoxic seizures, febrile delirium and breath-holding attacks, should be considered. The age of the child and degree of illness will further determine how the child is managed once the diagnosis of a FS is made. The first step would be to determine the source of infection. If this can be accurately determined, further investigations may not be indicated. Examination of the ear, throat, chest and nervous system is mandatory. A urine dip should be performed to rule out a urinary tract infection. A FS is not an indication for routine blood tests, and they should only be performed if a specific indication exists. A decision needs to be made on whether a lumbar puncture is indicated, and this will be determined by the suspected source of infection. If meningitis or encephalitis is suspected, a lumbar puncture should be performed unless contraindicated. In the older child (above two years of age), the clinical diagnosis of meningeal irritation may be easier to make. In the absence of suggestive signs (such as neck stiffness and photophobia), with a clear alternative source of infection, a lumbar puncture would not be necessary. However, in the younger child, particularly less than one year of age, the diagnosis may be difficult on clinical grounds due to the subtlety with which they may present. Poor feeding, irritability and lethargy may be signs of meningitis, and in such a scenario, a lumbar puncture should be strongly considered. There is no evidence that EEG, done at the time of presentation or up to a month later, has any prognostic or diagnostic benefit. This is the case for simple and complex FSs. It should therefore not be routinely performed. A FS may herald the onset of an epileptic disorder, such as Dravet syndrome, in which case an EEG will be performed. However, the suspicion of such syndromes is raised after multiple febrile or afebrile seizures. In the absence of abnormal neurological findings, there is no need for neuro-imaging for either simple or complex FSs. In the presence of neurological abnormalities, a non-urgent magnetic resonance image (MRI) should be organized.

Immediate management to terminate the seizure is indicated if the seizure is prolonged. Treatment should be given if the seizure lasts longer than five minutes. Rectal diazepam or buccal midazolam at a dose of 0.5 mg/kg is effective at terminating seizures. Midazolam may also be given intranasally. They are the drugs of choice in the primary care setting due to the likelihood of not having intravenous access. In a study comparing the two benzodiazepines in children aged six months and older attending hospital, buccal midazolam was found to be more effective than rectal diazepam in terminating the seizure within 10 minutes for at least an hour (McIntyre et al.). If the seizure is not terminated within 10 minutes of delivery of the drug, or the seizure recurs, then an ambulance should be called to organize hospital admission. Long-term management is centred on parent reassurance and explanation of the condition.

The mother in this case enquires about prophylaxis. As discussed earlier, evidence in favour of regular antipyretic prescribing to prevent the recurrence of a FS is lacking. Nevertheless, antipyretics should be used to make the child more comfortable. Long-term anticonvulsant treatment has been used in the past but is no longer recommended due to the lack of evidence of its effectiveness in reducing the risk of a recurrence or reducing the risk of epilepsy. Coupled with an unfavourable side effect profile, it is not usually difficult to convince parents against the use of regular antiepileptic medication. Since the use of regular preventative medication has fallen out of use, intermittent use of preventative benzodiazepines has gained some favour. Studies have shown intermittent use of diazepam, during a febrile episode, to be effective in preventing a recurrence of FS. Side effects associated with diazepam use in such a manner included lethargy, irritability and ataxia, with up to a third of children affected in one study. A discussion with the parent should revolve around whether preventing a recurrence is necessary or not. Risk factors for an increased risk of recurrence include:

- First FS below the age of 18 months
- History of FSs in a first-degree relative
- Shorter duration of fever (<1 h) prior to seizure onset
- Seizure occurring at relatively lower temperature (35% within one year with a recorded temperature of 38.3 °C, reducing to 13% with a temperature of 40.6 °C or higher)
- Multiple seizures occurring in the same febrile episode

In the absence of these features, parents may wish not to embark on benzodiazepine prophylaxis.

Learning Tip

"The single biggest problem with communication is the illusion that it has taken place." This quote of George Bernard Shaw succinctly expresses the importance of good communication skills. Communicating and predicting outcomes is, arguably, all we do as general practitioners. Day in, day out, one consultation after the other, we rely on our communication skills to extract the relevant information from our patients, make them feel at ease and predict the course of their ailment, hoping that their recovery will coincide with the treatment we have suggested. We all will have come across instances where a breakdown in communication can derail the entire course of a consultation. Despite all the advances in medicine, good communication skills remain indispensable to a successful consultation. Having all the knowledge about the condition means little if it cannot be communicated in a simple and comprehensible manner.

AKT PREPARATION

Options for questions 26–30:

a. West's syndrome
b. Breath-holding attacks
c. Sandifer syndrome

d. Absence seizures
e. Benign rolandic epilepsy
f. Angelman syndrome
g. Pavus nocturnus
h. Panic attacks

Questions 26–30 are about children presenting with a "funny turn". From the list above, choose the most appropriate diagnosis that fits the clinical presentation. Each option may be used once, more than once or not at all.

26. A five-year-old girl is seen in the epilepsy clinic. She is noted to have coarse features. Mum tells you that she has sudden outbursts of unprovoked laughter and is fascinated by running water.

27. An eight-year-old boy presents with tingling in his mouth, lips and gums on waking in the morning. On a few occasions, dad has noticed his speech to be unclear.

28. A two-year-old boy passes out after he is told off. Mum says that he was crying and became red in the face prior to passing out. She does not report any abnormal jerking, and he regained consciousness within a minute.

29. Which of the following statements regarding retinoblastoma is false?

   a. Retinoblastoma is the commonest primary ocular tumour in children.
   b. Retinoblastoma is a life-threatening condition with approximately 50% mortality rate in the first year in the UK.
   c. The diagnosis of retinoblastoma is delayed in most cases.
   d. A new-onset strabismus may be a sign of a retinoblastoma.
   e. Children with an inherited form of retinoblastoma are at an increased risk of developing non-ocular cancers later in life.

30. Which of the following signs is usually positive in Marfan's syndrome?

   a. Steinberlg's sign
   b. Gower's sign
   c. Rovsing's sign
   d. Scarf sign
   e. Murphy's sign

BIBLIOGRAPHY

American Academy of Pediatrics. Provisional Committee on Quality Improvement, Subcommittee on Febrile Seizures. Practice parameter: The neurodiagnostic evaluation of the child with a first simple febrile seizure. *Pediatrics* 1996 May; **97**(5):769–72; discussion 773–5.

Barr DGD, Crofton PM, Goel KM. Disorders of bone, joints and connective tissue. In: Campbell AGM, McIntosh N. *Forfar & Arneil's Textbook of Pediatrics.* Churchill Livingstone. 1998. P. 1544–615.

Berg AT, Shinnar S, Hauser WA *et al.* A prospective study of recurrent febrile seizures. *N Engl J Med* 1992; **327**:1122–27.

Brown JK, Minns RA. Disorders of the central nervous system. Surgical paediatrics. In: Campbell AGM, McIntosh N. *Forfar & Arneil's Textbook of Pediatrics.* Churchill Livingstone; 1998. P. 641–846.

Butros LJ, Abramson DH, Dunkel IJ. Delayed diagnosis of retinoblastoma: Analysis of degree, cause, and potential consequences. *Pediatrics* 2002 Mar; **109**(3):E45.

Cuestas E. Is routine EEG helpful in the management of complex febrile seizures? *Arch Dis Child* 2004; **89**:290.

El-Radhi SA, Barry W. Do antipyretics prevent febrile convulsions? *Arch Dis Child* 2003; **88**:641–2.

Joint Working Group of the Research Unit of the Royal College of Physicians and the British Paediatric Association. Guidelines for the management of convulsions with fever. *BMJ* 1991; **303**(6803):634–6.

McIntyre J, Robertson S, Norris E *et al.* Safety and efficacy of buccal midazolam versus rectal diazepam for emergency treatment of seizures in children: A randomised controlled trial. *Lancet* 2005; **366**:205–10.

Rosman NP, Colton T, Labazzo J *et al.* A controlled trial of diazepam administered during febrile illnesses to prevent recurrence of febrile seizures. *N Engl J Med* 1993; **329**:79–84.

Sadleir LG, Scheffer IE. Febrile seizures. *BMJ* 2007; **334**(7588):307–11.

Srinivasan J, Wallace KA, Scheffer IE. Febrile seizures. *Aust Fam Physician* 2005; **34**(12):1021–25.

Stuijvenberg M, Derksen-Lubsen G, Steyerberg EW *et al.* Randomized, controlled trial of ibuprofen syrup administered during febrile illnesses to prevent febrile seizure recurrences. *Pediatrics* 1998; **102**(5):e51.

Waruiru C, Appleton R. Febrile seizures: An update. *Arch Dis Child* 2004; **89**:751–6.

Yun J, Li Y, Xu CT, Pan BR. Epidemiology and Rb1 gene of retinoblastoma. *Int J Ophthalmol* 2011; **4**(1):103–9.

7

Case 7: Acne

A 15-year-old boy comes to see you in your clinic. He is captain of the school basketball team. You note that he came to see your colleague three weeks ago complaining about his skin. Acne was diagnosed, and a topical antibiotic was prescribed. He is clutching a piece of paper as he walks in today. He tells you that the antibiotic gel that he was prescribed did nothing for his skin. A friend of his saw a private dermatologist, who had prescribed him a drug that had immediately cured his acne. He has the name of the drug scribbled on this piece of paper: isotretinoin. He requests that he be prescribed this for his acne also, as he is suffering from a lack of self-confidence due to the state of his skin. Close examination of the skin reveals four to five comedones scattered around the forehead. No other lesions are seen elsewhere, and his back and chest are also clear. The only other noticeable thing in his notes is that he was under the care of the paediatric mental health team two years ago due to self-harming behaviour after the death of his father from a myocardial infarction at the age of 50.

Which of the following statements is true?

a. He should be advised that his acne is not severe enough to warrant any treatment and that he should wait for it to settle on its own.
b. Isotretinoin is contraindicated in him due to his past history of mental health problems.
c. Isotretinoin may lead to permanent remission of the acne.
d. Isotretinoin therapy may lower triglyceride levels.
e. Women who fall pregnant on isotretinoin should be reassured that data from animal studies suggest that it is safe to take the drug up to the end of the first trimester.

DOI: 10.1201/9781003449737-8

ANSWER

c is correct

Acne is amongst the commonest skin conditions affecting teenagers. It is a cause of considerable anxiety and psychological morbidity amongst sufferers. It is not uncommon in clinical practice to find some teenagers to be completely unbothered by severe widespread acne and others to be extremely distressed by a few spots scattered here and there. It is therefore important to consider the impact the condition has on the patient whilst formulating a management plan. By a series of questionnaires, Mallon et al. demonstrated that sufferers from severe acne may suffer from similar levels of psychological morbidity as diabetes, asthma and epilepsy sufferers. It is therefore important that the patient's plight is not trivialized despite the fact he may be suffering from mild acne.

Acne is characterized by the presence of comedones, which are non-inflammatory follicular lesions. The follicle may be open (blackheads) or closed (whiteheads). They may be the only lesions present or may be accompanied by inflamed papules, cysts and pustules. The more severe the acne, the larger, deeper and more inflamed are the lesions. In severe cases, deep nodular lesions may develop, which are filled with mucopurulent material and are more likely to scar. In a rare form of acne, acne conglobata, these nodules may interconnect and require drainage, resulting in an exceptionally severe form of disease.

Treatment of acne is determined by the severity of disease and may be topical or by oral medication. Some people may mistake blackheads for dirt and be excessive in their attempts to clean these lesions. They should be advised that blackheads are just open follicles, full of sebum and dead cells. Their black colour is due to the oxidization of the melanin pigment. Excessive cleaning may result in skin irritation, making them less likely to tolerate some of the topical treatments discussed below. Once a day gentle scrubbing to remove dead cells and avoidance of the application of oily substances (such as make-up) to the skin should help with simple comedonal lesions. However, clinicians who deal with acne on a daily basis will know that rarely will most teenagers be satisfied just with advice, as most will seek some form of treatment to help with the lesions.

TOPICAL TREATMENT

In mild-to-moderate acne, it is appropriate to start with topical treatment. Topical treatment may consist of the following:

- Antibacterials
- Retinoids
- Keratolytics
- Combination therapy

Antibacterials are targeted against *Propionibacterium acnes*, the chief colonizer of the pilosebaceous unit. Topical preparations of erythromycin and clindamycin may be used to treat inflammatory lesions. As with all topical treatments, skin irritation may occur. The primary problem with topical antibacterials is the development of antibacterial resistance. This is likely to demonstrate itself as a reduced clinical response to the topical preparations. To prevent resistance from developing, concomitant use with oral antibiotics and unnecessarily long uninterrupted courses should be avoided. Another way of avoiding the development of resistance is the simultaneous use of the topical **keratolytic agents**, which break down keratin and hence have exfoliative and comedolytic properties. Benzoyl peroxide is a powerful oxidizing agent with antibacterial activity as well. When used with erythromycin, it has been shown to reduce the development of antibacterial resistance (Harkaway et al.). Hence, combination treatment with the two or courses of topical antibacterial therapy broken with benzoyl peroxide use may be an effective way of treating acne whilst reducing the risk of the development of resistant bacterial strains. Azelaic acid is another keratolytic agent with antibacterial activity, which has the advantage of being less likely to cause skin irritation when compared with benzoyl peroxide. **Topical retinoids**, which are vitamin A derivatives, have anti-comedonal and anti-inflammatory properties. Retinoids interact with retinoid receptors and thereby effect the proliferation and differentiation of epithelial cells. This encourages exfoliation and reduced comedonal formation. Their contact with mucous membranes and peeling skin should be avoided, as should exposure to ultraviolet light post-application. Hence, they are usually applied at night. They are contraindicated in pregnant women due the risk of embryopathy. Adapalene 0.1%, a topical retinoid, has been shown to be effective when used in combination with benzoyl peroxide 2.5% when compared with using either one of them alone. This combination has been shown to have an early onset of action and to be effective against treating inflammatory and non-inflammatory lesions (Keating). Topical treatments should be prescribed for at least three to six months in order to see the full impact of their effect.

ORAL TREATMENT

Oral options for males include antibiotics and retinoids. In females, hormonal treatment is another option. Oral antibiotics with evidence of benefit include erythromycin and the tetracyclines: tetracycline, oxytetracycline, doxycycline, minocycline and lymecycline. Resistance to erythromycin is becoming more common. If there is a lack of response or a flare-up whilst taking treatment, an alternative antibiotic should be sought. Tetracycline or oxytetracycline will generally be used first line. They are used in twice-daily regimes, and it is appropriate to wait for three months for a response. If adequate response is seen, treatment should continue for at least six months. In some cases, it may be necessary to continue for two years. They are taken on an empty stomach, with particular avoidance of milk, which reduces their absorption. A lack of adequate response warrants a switch to one of the other tetracyclines. Doxycycline and lymecycline have the advantage of once-daily dosing: 100 mg and 408 mg daily, respectively. Minocycline is given at a dose of

100 mg once a day or 50 mg twice daily. All tetracyclines carry the risk of causing drug-induced lupus erythematosus, but the risk with minocycline is the highest. Tetracyclines are deposited in growing bone and teeth and hence should not be given to children under the age of 12 or during pregnancy and lactation. If there is a lack of response to two different antibiotics, and a switch to oral retinoids is being considered, trimethoprim may be considered as a third-line antibiotic. Its use in the context of acne is unlicensed, but at a dose of 300 mg twice daily, it has been shown to be effective and reasonably safe (Cunliffe et al.). Prolonged use of trimethoprim has been associated with marrow suppression (not as likely as when used in combination with sulfamethoxazole).

Isotretinoin, the oral retinoid licensed for use in acne, is the drug that the patient seems to be interested in due to the effects it had on his friend. Isotretinoin is more effective than the above-mentioned treatment options but also has the potential for more serious side effects. Isotretinoin not only stunts the growth of *P. acnes*; it also reduces the size of the pilosebaceous unit and encourages normal follicular keratinization. It is therefore effective against comedonal and inflammatory disease. The list of potential side effects is large, but dryness of eyes, mucosa and skin should be warned against. Infections of the skin and mucosa should be monitored for. It has also been associated with raised triglyceride levels and raised serum cholesterol with a drop in high density lipoprotein levels. This may be significant in this case due to the young age at which his father suffered from a myocardial infarction. Cholesterol and triglyceride levels are routinely measured before and during isotretinoin therapy. Another important consideration is the association between isotretinoin use and depression, necessitating a mental health review during follow-up appointments (Azoulay et al.). Although a concern, the patient's history of depression is not an absolute contraindication to the use of isotretinoin. Although isotretinoin therapy is initiated by dermatologists, it is important to be aware of the potential complications of treatment so that they may be readily recognized in primary care. Since the severity perceived by the patient is also important in how acne is managed, isotretinoin should be considered in patients if they are extremely distressed by it. This patient should be made aware of the potential side effects of the drug and the existence of alternatives which he has not yet tried and which are likely to produce the desired effect due to the mild nature of his condition. Regular reviews may be necessary to reassure him and monitor the effects of therapy.

Learning Tip

Managing patient expectations can be a complicated aspect of the doctor–patient consultation. Patients may have pre-conceived ideas about their condition and the subsequent treatment or referrals that may or may not be needed. This conflict can be compounded if the patient receives conflicting advice from different clinicians. It is important to communicate with the patient in a manner that they can easily understand and show empathy towards their concerns. A relationship based on trust with the patient goes a long way in ensuring that the doctor and the patient reach a common understanding of the problem and how to manage it.

AKT PREPARATION

Options for questions 31–35:

a. Impetigo
b. Molluscum contagiosum
c. Pityriasis rosea
d. Erythema toxicum neonatorum
e. Papular acrodermatitis of childhood
f. Pediculosis capitis
g. Acrodermatitis enteropathica
h. Erythema marginatum
i. Pityriasis versicolor

Questions 31–35 refer to children presenting with a rash. Choose the most likely diagnosis for questions 31–35 from the list above. Each option may be used once, more than once or not at all.

31. A 12-year-old boy is seen with a widespread rash consisting of oval macules spread in a "fir tree pattern" over the trunk. He is systemically well and reports a single lesion appearing on his neck three days prior to the widespread rash.

32. A six-month-old girl with cystic fibrosis presents with an erythematous, crusted rash around the mouth and nose. Blood tests reveal negligible zinc levels.

33. A three-year-old girl presents with a crop of pearly white, dome-shaped lesions just under her right armpit. Mum thinks they may have appeared since she started swimming at the local swimming pool.

34. Which of the following statements regarding haemangiomas is/are true?

    a. Haemangiomas are benign proliferative tumours of endothelial cells.
    b. They are usually present at birth, after which they go through a slow growth phase.
    c. They should always be treated upon identification due to the risk of haemorrhagic bleed.
    d. Oral or intralesional steroids may be used to help slow their growth.
    e. Sturge–Weber syndrome describes a haemangioma of the face associated with a lesion on the ipsilateral meninges and cerebral cortex.

35. Congenital absence of the canal of Schlemm may result in which condition of the eye?

    a. Buphthalmos
    b. Infantile macular degeneration
    c. Congenital obstruction of the nasolacrimal duct
    d. Meibomian cyst
    e. Entropion

BIBLIOGRAPHY

Azoulay L, Blais L, Koren G *et al.* Isotretinoin and the risk of depression in patients with acne vulgaris: A case-crossover study. *J Clin Psychiatry* 2008 Apr; **69**(4):526–32.

Cant JS. Disorders of the eye. In: Campbell AGM, McIntosh N. *Forfar & Arneil's Textbook of Pediatrics.* Churchill Livingstone; 1998. P. 1649–78.

Cunliffe WJ, Aldana OL, Goulden V. Oral trimethoprim: A relatively safe and successful third-line treatment for acne vulgaris. *Br J Dermatol* 1999 Oct; **141**(4):757–8.

Goulden V. Guidelines for the management of acne vulgaris in adolescents. *Paediatr Drugs* 2003; **5**(5):301–13.

Harkaway KS, McGinley KJ, Foglia AN *et al.* Antibiotic resistance patterns in coagulase-negative staphylococci after treatment with topical erythromycin, benzoyl peroxide, and combination therapy. *Br Dermatol* 1992; **126**:586–90.

Healy E, Simpson N. Acne vulgaris. *BMJ* 1994; **308**:831–3.

James WD. Acne. *N Engl J Med* 2005; **352**:1463–72.

Keating GM. Adapalene 0.1%/benzoyl peroxide 2.5% gel: A review of its use in the treatment of acne vulgaris in patients aged ≥ 12 years. *Am J Clin Dermatol* 2011 Dec 1; **12**(6):407–20.

Mallon E, Newton JN, Klassen A *et al.* The quality of life in acne: A comparison with general medical conditions using generic questionnaires. *Br J Dermatol* 1999; **140**(4):672–6.

Motamedi M, Chehade A, Sanghera R, Grewal P. A clinician's guide to topical retinoids. *J Cutan Med Surg* 2022 Jan–Feb; **26**(1):71–78.

Rogers M, Barnetson RSC. Diseases of the skin. In: Campbell AGM, McIntosh N. *Forfar & Arneil's Textbook of Pediatrics.* Churchill Livingstone; 1998. P. 1616–48.

Starkey E, Shahidullah H. Propranolol for infantile haemangiomas: A review. *Arch Dis Child* 2011 Sep; **96**(9):890–3.

Stulberg DL, Wolfrey J. Pityriasis rosea. *Am Fam Physician* 2004 Jan 1; **69**(1):87–91.

8

Case 8: Outbreak

You are assigned to the clinical rounds at a local immigration detention centre. On arrival, you are given the list of patients you are required to see. You notice there are two individuals with a fever and rash amongst the other patients. You ask to see the first of these patients, who is a six-year-old Afghani boy. The child has had a fever for three days with a runny nose and eyes. Last night he broke out in a rash on his face, which has now spread to the rest of the body. Although systemically well, he has a high fever and is slightly irritable. Examination of his mouth reveals tiny white spots, which you suspect to be Koplik spots. You also note a widespread maculopapular rash that has coalesced in places. The second patient with a similar rash is the child's older sister. The vaccination history of both is unavailable. You suspect that both children are suffering from measles.

Which of the following statements is/are true?

a. Measles is a notifiable disease in the UK.
b. Measles is no longer infectious once the typical rash appears.
c. Measles, mumps and rubella (MMR) vaccine is highly effective at preventing measles.
d. There is no need to isolate the children until the diagnosis of measles has been confirmed, as a similar rash can be present in other viral infections.
e. Measles infection, having previously received the vaccine, is termed "breakthrough measles" and is associated with a higher level of infectivity.

DOI: 10.1201/9781003449737-9

ANSWER

a and c are true

The highly unpredictable and variable nature of clinical scenarios encountered in general practice is a well-recognized phenomenon known all too well to those who practise it on a regular basis. However, even in the arbitrary randomness, there is a sense of familiarity, a perception of order, which allows the practitioner to discern any anomalies that may threaten to disrupt the orderly pattern of an unpredictable clinic. Being, quite literally, on the front line gives a first-hand feel of any unusual surge of alternative presentations. A sudden increase in children presenting with a fever and a rash in the winter or an unexpected rise in demand for inhalers during the hay fever season is usually immediately felt at the coalface of general practice, making it an ideal set-up for surveillance of unusual outbreaks.

An outbreak of any scale of a transmissible infection brings a unique set of challenges and responsibilities for a primary care physician. This novelty was at its most obvious during the recent Covid-19 pandemic: a truly global event associated with unprecedented paralysis of the world economy and limitation of movement of people. Sudden outbreaks such as those in our case above or the Covid-19 pandemic can induce fear not only in

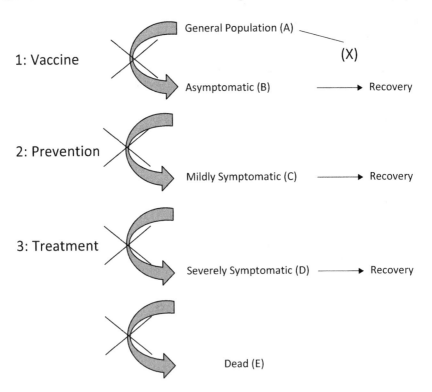

Figure 8.1 The outbreak: A runaway train.

the general population but also in health care professionals charged with dealing with its consequences. Covid-19 carried the added fear of an unknown illness with no prior immunity and a fearsome reputation for severe consequences.

This case looks at concepts that need to be considered in the management of an outbreak of an infectious illness. These ideas will inform our decisions on how best to act and manage a situation such as the one in the case above. Figure 8.1 gives the outbreak a visual form.

THE OUTBREAK: A RUNAWAY TRAIN

Think of the outbreak as a runaway train as it passes through point A. This train is heading towards its inevitable destination of death at E. To help devise an effective management strategy in this situation, we can divide those at risk into two categories:

- *The uninfected*: Those at A who are yet to embark on the train.
- *The infected*: Those who are already on the train from B to E.

THE UNINFECTED

The first aim is to determine what proportion of the people at A will end up starting the journey. This is crucially important, as it will ultimately determine the likely number of people who will end up at all of the other destinations in the flow diagram. In the case of a novel virus, such as Covid-19, the majority will have to get on the train at some point. When a certain proportion of the population have embarked on the runaway train, it will lose its potency and the capability to be able to pick up more passengers: a concept referred to as herd immunity. Due to incomplete medical records and people fleeing often dire circumstances, it would be safer to assume that most of the residents of the detention centre are susceptible to catching the virus and spreading it on.

A useful tool to determine at what rate people from the general population are boarding the train is known as the R value. In viral terms, this refers to the growth capacity of the virus. If a virus has an R value of 1, then it means that one infectious person, on average, will generate one new infection. In simple terms, it determines how many people one infected case can be expected to pass the infection on to. The higher the R value, the quicker the outbreak will grow. Pandemic flu has an R value of around 1 to 2, whereas measles, unmitigated by any protection, can have an R value of 20, resulting in explosive increases in the number of infections among susceptible populations. But, the R value is not an inherent value of the virus. It is determined by a number of factors that can be altered in order to alter the R value of the viral outbreak. A useful mnemonic to remember these factors, described by Adam Kucharski in his book *The Rules of Contagion*, is DOTS:

D = Duration for which the individual with the infection is infectious. If viral shedding is taking place over a longer time, it will give the individual a greater opportunity to spread the infection, giving the outbreak a high R value. In the case of measles, the infectious period usually starts four days before the rash appears and lasts for up to four days after the rash.

O = Opportunity to spread the infection. If the average number of social contacts per person per day in one subset of society is higher than in another, there will be a greater opportunity to spread the infection in the former and hence, a higher R value. The usually overcrowded nature of detention centres makes them more vulnerable to dramatically fast spread of infections.

T = Transmission probability. In the absence of herd immunity, the chance that each contact will transmit infection is higher, so there is a consequently higher R value.

S = Average susceptibility of the population. A population with poor uptake of vaccination or more immunocompromised patients is more likely to transmit the virus due to poorer immunity.

It becomes apparent that manipulating the different factors affecting the R value can change the rate of growth of the virus. Social distancing, quarantining, self-isolation and lockdowns are all methods deployed to reduce the risk of the spread of the virus by lowering the R value.

R values are not, however, relevant to just viruses and other infectious agents; R values can also be applied to the spreading of false information. The spread of false or incomplete information can induce panic by instilling fear in those exposed to any threat from an outbreak such as this. This phenomenon was particularly apparent during the recent Covid-19 pandemic. Many conspiracy theories and false cures were propagated through the internet and the use of social media. If one person forwards a message to 20 people, and each one of them forwards it to another 20 people (R value of 20), within 5 cycles, the message can reach more than 3 million people. Such a frightening capability to spread information can have a horrendous effect on health care services as the worried well increasingly seek reassurance, in some instances totally overwhelming the system.

THE INFECTED

As our train blasts through point A, it picks up people according to their exposure and susceptibilities such as age, co-morbidities, genetics and sex. The hope is that the majority of those who board the train are strong enough to be able to disembark at B. For them, the horrific train ride is barely noticeable, and most are unaware that they were ever on it. This could include patients who have previously been vaccinated against measles. Catching measles after being fully vaccinated against it is termed breakthrough measles and is associated with milder symptoms and a lower level of infectivity. In some cases, they may not even develop a rash. Some patients are unable to disembark at B and end up continuing the journey. For them, the ride is a slight inconvenience as they experience some of the discomforts of the journey as they disembark at C with no major ongoing sequelae. There are a few who unfortunately are unable to end the nightmare here. For them, the journey is a considerable inconvenience as they feel the full force of the horror of the journey. Yet, the majority will still have the strength and resilience to disembark at D. They may be scarred by the journey but will avoid its ultimate destination at E. In the case of measles, common complications include diarrhoea, otitis media and tracheobronchitis. Rarer, but more serious, complications include pneumonia, encephalitis and subacute sclerosing panencephalitis, the latter occurring many years after the initial infection and always leading to death.

The proportion of people ending up at E from all those who embark on the train at A is termed the mortality rate of the infectious agent. The mortality rate of measles is approximately 0.1%, whereas that of seasonal influenza can vary year on year depending on vaccine uptake and circulating strains. Improved outcomes can be sought out by disrupting the journey at various stages. The most desirable would be to prevent it at step 1, reducing the chances of people boarding the train in the first place. The highly infectious nature of measles can mean that a small decrease in the uptake of the MMR vaccine can lead to localized outbreaks. The Covid-19 pandemic ground the world to a halt until effective vaccines started to become available. Vaccines have always been subject to scrutiny and at times quite vitriolic negative campaigns, which can contribute to more frequent outbreaks of the conditions they are meant to suppress. Recently, declining vaccination rates have meant that a global increase in measles outbreaks has become a worrying reality.

No matter how successful the vaccine programme is, it is inevitable that people will continue to board the train, and therefore, it is desirable to develop treatment modalities to disrupt the journey at stages 2 and 3 as well. Prevention via good hygiene and mask usage and immune system enhancement strategies such as good nutrition, exercise and adequate sleep can help stop the train much earlier in the journey. Disease-specific treatments are the final roadblock one can put in the way to prevent the train from hurtling towards E. The detour towards X represents the undesirable mutation of viral strains, which can take outbreaks in unpredictable directions. Surveillance of outbreaks is of paramount importance to be able to identify mutated strains early so that preventative measures are put in place in a timely fashion.

Learning Tip

In the age of digital communication, medical information is increasingly shared and accessed by doctors and patients alike via social media forums (SMFs). Despite its benefits, the phenomenon brings with it unique challenges too. Patients may expect treatments that they may have heard of on SMFs, which may have little or no evidence supporting their use. Researching this may take a huge amount of time and effort on the part of the doctor. Doctors using SMFs also need to be aware of the ethical challenges such media present in terms of maintaining professionalism and confidentiality.

AKT PREPARATION

Options for questions 36–40:

a. Coxsackie group A virus
b. Parvovirus B19
c. Herpes simplex virus
d. Human herpes virus 6 (HHV-6)
e. Human papillomavirus (HPV)
f. Varicella zoster virus
g. Epstein–Barr virus
h. Mumps virus

From the options above, choose the most likely causative agent in the children presenting with viral illnesses in questions 36–40. Each option may be used once, more than once or not at all.

36. A 14-year-old boy presents with bilaterally enlarged parotid glands and a painful swollen right testicle.

37. A four-year-old girl presents with a sore throat, low-grade fever and small blisters on her hands and feet and inside the mouth.

38. A three-year-old boy develops a high temperature, runny nose and watery eyes. The temperature finally abates on the fourth day, and just as Mum thought he was improving, he breaks out in a pinkish rash on his torso, spreading to his arms and legs. The rash blanches on pressure and disappears after 48 hours.

39. Which of the following statements regarding vaccinations are true?

    a. Diphtheria, tetanus and pertussis (DTP) vaccine may be associated with an increased mortality from infections other than diphtheria, tetanus and pertussis in high-mortality areas.
    b. The child's response to a vaccine may differ depending on the vaccinations and infections they may have had in the past.
    c. The measles vaccine has been associated with a reduced mortality from infections other than measles.
    d. Vaccination of pregnant mothers with the pertussis vaccine to prevent neonatal infections is not recommended due to the risk of Arthus reactions.
    e. Vaccinating close household contacts of young infants against pertussis does not reduce the risk of pertussis acquisition by the infant.

40. Which of the following is a not a live vaccine?

   a. Measles
   b. Rubella
   c. Oral polio
   d. Rabies
   e. Rotavirus

BIBLIOGRAPHY

Amirthalingham G. Strategies to control pertussis in infants. *Arch Dis Child* 2013; **98**:552–5.

Deer B. How the case against the MMR vaccine was fixed. *BMJ* 2011; **342**:c5347.

Iacobucci G. Measles is now "an imminent threat" globally, WHO and CDC warn. *BMJ* 2022; **379**:o2844.

Knight S, Hayhoe B, Papanikitas A, Sajid I. Ethical issues in the use of online social media forums by GPs. *Br J Gen Pract* 2019 Apr;**69**(681):203–4.

Kucharski A. *The Rules of Contagion: Why Things Spread and Why They Stop.* Profile Books Ltd; 2020.

National Measles Guidelines. Public Health England. 2019 Nov. https://assets.publishing.service.gov.uk/government/uploads/system/uploads/attachment_data/file/849538/PHE_Measles_Guidelines.pdf

Pittet LF, Messina NL, Orsini F *et al*; BRACE Trial Consortium Group. Randomized trial of BCG vaccine to protect against Covid-19 in health care workers. *N Engl J Med* 2023 Apr 27; **388**(17):1582–1596.

Razaq S. It's the sun wot won it. *BJGP* 2023;**73**(727):78.

Shann F. The non-specific effects of vaccines. *Arch Dis Child* 2010; **95**:662–7.

9

Case 9: Statistics 1

A 44-year-old patient of yours, who is well known to you, presents with concerns regarding breast cancer. She has not noticed any changes in her breast but has found herself worrying a lot since a friend of hers recently died of the disease. She is aware that she is not entitled to a mammogram on the national screening programme but is able to get one through her private insurance as long as she gets a referral from a doctor. She asks you for the referral so she can get a mammogram at the local private hospital. You reluctantly agree and receive a report from the private hospital one week later that the mammogram has found a suspicious lesion suggestive of breast cancer. It is now your duty to call the patient and inform her of the results. The breast unit informs you that the testing equipment has a sensitivity of 92% and a specificity of 95%. (The prevalence of breast cancer in this age group is around 1.5%.)

Which of the following statements is/are true?

a. The patient has a greater than 90% probability of having breast cancer after a positive test.
b. The patient has a greater than 50% but less than 90% probability of having breast cancer after a positive test.
c. A specificity of 95% means that 5% of the results will be false negatives.
d. The high sensitivity and specificity of the test ensure that the final results are highly accurate.
e. None of the above.

DOI: 10.1201/9781003449737-10

ANSWER

e is correct

Homer's *Odyssey* tells the story of Odysseus' perilous journey home: a voyage full of wondrous horrors such as Scylla, a six-headed monster, and Charybdis, a whirlpool capable of swallowing entire ships. When the crew disobey Odysseus and slaughter the cattle of the Sun, Zeus, as punishment, unleashes a massive storm, sinking the ship and killing all the crew members. Odysseus barely survives by hanging on to the root of a fig tree, *rhizikon* in Classical Greek. It is believed that the word *risk* originates from this precarious state of Odysseus. Or perhaps it has its roots in the Arabic word *rizq*, referring to the predetermined subsistence provided by God, alluding to the inescapable element of fate.

Defining and dealing with risk, such as in the case above, is the absolute bread and butter of the primary care physician's daily work. However, it is rarely conceptualized into a case with actual numbers and statistical terms in our day-to-day work. We will almost certainly rely on heuristics: short cuts that allow us to resolve complex pieces of information based on previous experiences and intuition. Whether relying on these heuristics allows us to reach an appropriate answer or not is a question this case hopes to elucidate.

This is one of those cases that some may completely breeze through, whilst others may have difficulty in visualizing the information in a way that allows a coherent assessment of the risk to be calculated. We can work through the case as follows.

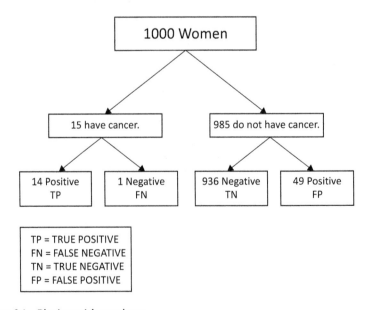

Figure 9.1 Playing with numbers.

The prevalence of breast cancer (which is the same as pre-test probability) in the fourth decade of life is approximately 1.5% (Howlader). So, in a sample of 1000 women (with no other symptoms, as in the patient in the case above), 15 women will have cancer, and 985 women will be cancer-free. The sensitivity of the test will determine the percentage of patients with the disease who are correctly identified (true positives). The specificity of the test will determine the percentage of patients without the disease who are correctly identified (true negatives). This can be shown, for ease, as in Figure 9.1.

As the figure shows, there are a total of 63 positive test results, of which only 14 are true positives. Hence, after a positive result, the probability that the abnormality detected actually represents a breast cancer is 14/63 = 22% (TP/TP + FP).

In statistical terms, this is known as the positive predictive value (PPV) of the test: 22% of those who test positive in the scenario above will actually have breast cancer. The other 78% will unfortunately endure additional stress and investigations until subsequent investigations rule out disease in them. The decision to proceed with a mammogram in this scenario does not seem like a sensible one anymore. The negative predictive value (NPV) of the test in this case is quite high at >99% (TN/TN + FN). Had the result been negative, it would have been highly reassuring.

The low predictive value of the test in this scenario often comes as a surprise to most clinicians, as a positive test result coupled with a respectably good test with high sensitivity and specificity intuitively suggests that the final result is highly accurate. However, this is due to what the economic journalist Tim Harford calls premature enumeration. Rather than approach the data with a degree of curiosity and scepticism, we tend to take the simple and easier explanation, which allows us to avoid uncomfortable mathematical gymnastics.

The reason why the positive predictive value seems to be so poor in this scenario, despite an acceptably accurate test, can be summarized as the context in which the patient presents, or in statistical terms, the pre-test probability (in this case, described as the prevalence). The prevalence of breast cancer in the fourth decade of life is thankfully quite low. A highly sensitive test is, therefore, likely to correctly identify most of the patients who have breast cancer. However, for the test result to be reliably interpreted, it needs to have a low false positive rate (FPR). The more false positive results there are, the lower the positive predictive value of the test will be. The FPR is a function of the specificity of the test; a test that is 100% specific will generate no false positives. The reliability of a test that is anything less than 100% specific will be dependent on the pre-test probability. The two scenarios below aim to demonstrate this in simple terms.

Imagine condition X. A test used for the detection of condition X has a sensitivity of 90% and a specificity of 95%. The results of testing for condition X in the two scenarios below will be presented in tabular form.

SCENARIO 1

Condition X has a prevalence of 60%.

Of 1000 people, 600 will have condition X, and 400 will not.

	Disease positive	Disease negative
Test positive	540 (TP)	20 (FP)
Test negative	60 (FN)	380 (TN)

PPV = TP/TP + FP = 540/560 = 96%

NPV = TN/TN + FN = 380/440 = 86%

SCENARIO 2

Condition X has a prevalence of 5%.

Of 1000 people, 50 will have condition X, and 950 will not.

	Disease positive	Disease negative
Test positive	45 (TP)	48 (FP)
Test negative	5 (FN)	902 (TN)

PPV = TP/TP + FP = 45/93 = 48%

NPV = TN/TN + FN = 902/907 = 99%

As is fairly clear from these two scenarios, the same test for the same condition has a significantly different PPV depending on the prevalence of the condition in the population in whom the test is being carried out. This is further demonstrated in the table below (the sensitivity and specificity of the test are 90% and 95%, respectively). Different clinicians may have different views regarding the cut-off at which the test loses its usefulness in terms of being able to accurately predict the presence of disease.

Prevalence	PPV	NPV
1%	15%	>99%
10%	67%	99%
20%	82%	97%
50%	95%	90%

In practical terms, this demonstrates the applicability of the test relevant to the clinical setting in which it is carried out. The dependability of a test for correctly identifying women presenting with suspicious breast lumps to a breast clinic (where the pre-test probability is high) will be different from the same test being used in asymptomatic women as a screening tool (where the pre-test probability will be low). Ignorance of this simple concept was displayed during the conversations surrounding the diagnosis of Covid-19 during the pandemic in the UK. At one point (when the prevalence of the virus in the community was stable at 0.1%), the government announced plans to carry out 10 million tests a day: the undeniably ambitious target termed "Operation Moonshot". With the stable prevalence of 0.1%, even a test with 99% sensitivity and 99% specificity would only yield a PPV of 9%, realization of which, perhaps, contributed to the idea being shelved fairly rapidly!

Learning Tip

Managing medical uncertainty can be a hugely challenging hurdle to the effective practice of medicine. One may employ various techniques to help with this challenge, but statistics offer one obvious solution. As the saying by Dr Theodore Woodward goes, "When you hear hoofbeats, think of horses, not zebras." We should think of statistics as our friend. One of the common reasons for uncertainty experienced by trainees and less experienced doctors is the over-worrying about missing the rarer diagnosis. This could be a leftover from medical school, where the student who correctly identifies the less than 1 in 100,000 eponymous syndrome based on a historically described triad named after a famous doctor from the past wins all the plaudits! In primary care, being overly keen to look for the most unlikely condition is likely to open a Pandora's Box that is likely to do more harm than good for the patient and enhance the clinician's sense of dread around medical uncertainty.

AKT PREPARATION

Options for questions 41–45:

a. 5%
b. 10%
c. 20%
d. 25%
e. 40%
f. 50%
g. 97.5%
h. 99%
i. None of the above

For questions 41–45, pick the correct answer from the options above. Each option may be used once, more than once or not at all.

41. A trial estimates that the sensitivity of the Rinne tuning fork test for detecting conductive hearing loss is 60% and the specificity is 80%. What would be the test's positive predictive value in a population with a 10% prevalence of conductive hearing loss?

42. A new test on the market aims to improve the diagnosis of prostate cancer. It is tested on 800 patients with known prostate cancer and is found to be positive in all but 20 patients. What is the specificity of this test?

43. Calculate the negative predictive value of a new malaria test (to the nearest whole number) that correctly identifies 810 people without disease. The test sample had 1000 patients, of whom 100 were known to have malaria at the time of the test. The sensitivity of the test is calculated to be 90%.

44. Which of the following statements regarding *p-value* is/are true?

    a. A *p-value* greater than 0.05 means that the null hypothesis is correct.
    b. A *p-value* less than 0.05 implies clinical importance of the parameters being measured.
    c. The smaller the *p-value*, the larger the effect, suggesting greater clinical significance.
    d. A *p-value* of less than 0.05 implies that the null hypothesis has a less than 5% chance of being rejected even though it is true.
    e. A *p-value* greater than 0.05 cannot be considered significant.

45. Which of the following statements regarding different types of research methods is/are false?

    a. Cross-sectional studies are used to determine prevalence.
    b. The efficiency of a prospective cohort study increases with increasing incidence of the studied outcome.
    c. A prospective cohort study must have an external control group in order to be able to analyse the difference from the study group.
    d. A retrospective cohort study is usually cheaper and quicker if the data is available.
    e. Prospective cohort studies can be hampered by the loss of participants to follow-up.

BIBLIOGRAPHY

Dahiru TP. Value, a true test of statistical significance? A cautionary note. *Ann Ib Postgrad Med* 2008 Jun; **6**(1):21–6.

Gigerenzer G. *Reckoning with Risk.* Penguin Press; 2002.

Harford T. *How to Make the World Add Up: Ten Rules for Thinking Differently about Numbers.* Bridge Street Press; 2020.

Howlader N, Noone AM, Krapcho M *et al.* (eds.). *SEER Cancer Statistics Review, 1975–2017.* National Cancer Institute; Apr 2020. https://seer.cancer.gov/csr/1975_2017/, based on November 2019 SEER data submission, posted to the SEER website.

Kwak S. Are only *p*-values less than 0.05 significant? A *p*-value greater than 0.05 is also significant! *J Lipid Atheroscler* 2023 May; **12**(2):89–95.

Mann CJ. Observational research methods. Research design II: Cohort, cross-sectional and case-control studies. *Emerg Med J* 2003; **20**:54–60.

Razaq S. Moonshot or shot in the dark? *BJGP Life* 2020 Sept 18. https://bjgplife.com/moonshot-or-shot-in-the-dark/

Razaq S. Reasoning with risk. *BJGP Life* 2020 Oct 28. https://bjgplife.com/reasoning-with-risk/

10

Case 10: Statistics 2

As the rush finally settles on a Friday afternoon on-call session, the receptionist calls that an anxious 28-year-old woman would like to discuss her blood results with you. She received a text from the surgery saying that she needs to urgently come in for review. You ask the receptionist to sit the patient in the waiting room whilst you look through the patient's notes. She saw your colleague two days ago. It is noted that she was seen with a swollen R calf, which was mildly tender. Your colleague had put "deep vein thrombosis (DVT) possible but unlikely" down in the notes and organized for a D-dimer blood test to be done. The result had come back as 880 ng/mL (laboratory cut-off for normal is 750 ng/mL). Your colleague had tried to contact the patient by phone, but having failed in doing so, sent an urgent text stating that her blood test was positive, and she should make an urgent appointment. As you call the patient in, she asks you in a state of panic whether she has a clot.

Which of the following statements is/are false?

a. With low suspicion of disease, D-dimer was a useful test in this case to help rule out a DVT.
b. The patient should be reassured that the test is only marginally positive, so her swollen, painful calf is not likely due to a DVT.
c. Wells score can be used to determine the pre-test probability of a DVT.
d. The patient should be referred for a compression duplex ultrasound, as it is the primary test for diagnosing a DVT.
e. Anticoagulation, unless strongly contraindicated, should be started in the patient until a DVT can be ruled out.

ANSWER

b is false

This case, in many ways, will build on some of the concepts we encountered in the previous one. This clinical scenario will not be too unfamiliar to many GPs: interpreting a result based on another clinician's judgement. Other, somewhat annoying, iterations of the above case could include:

- A letter from the local orthopaedic consultant, who saw your patient three days ago with an elbow fracture. The patient had some routine bloods, the potassium level was slightly elevated at 6.1 mmol/L and the consultant would like you to manage as you would see appropriate.
- A letter from the local accident and emergency department, who saw your patient with musculoskeletal chest pain but wanted to report a slightly elevated troponin for consideration in the ongoing management of the patient.
- A letter from the radiology department, who, after reviewing a chest X-ray carried out on a patient in the accident and emergency department having attended with chest injury after a road traffic accident, would like to inform you of a lesion in the left base, which is difficult to characterize.

These cases, and countless similar others that are frequently encountered in primary care, raise an important question: what do test results actually mean in the absence of a clinical context? If all patients presenting to the casualty department with chest pain have a troponin and D-dimer level checked prior to a history and examination, what value do the results actually hold? What degree of importance should be given to a positive result in this scenario if the diagnosis based on history and examination was costochondritis?

The previous case demonstrates that tests in themselves can be flawed; they can detect disease when it is absent and miss disease when it is present. In practical terms, this can result in a huge amount of distress for a patient, manifested as unnecessary worry, futile and invasive investigations, and false reassurance. Individual responsibility is rarely challenged on multiple unnecessary invasive investigations. Similarly, the unnecessary distress caused to patients through false positives cannot be objectivized. Conversely, however, false reassurance, ultimately, can lead to delayed diagnosis and catastrophic consequences. If this does not affect the responsible clinician litigiously, it certainly affects them psychologically with guilt and a sense of under-achievement. This sequence of thought processes, unfortunately, leads to continued over-investigation through tests, the rationale for which can often be poorly thought out.

But, is there a way of bringing more objectivity and hence, more confidence to the process of decision making? As clinicians, we are constantly reviewing the information we receive from our patients, which impacts on our understanding of what the problem may be. Our differential diagnosis list constantly changes as more and more information is extracted through either history taking, examination or test results. This process has an underlying mathematical correlation, which we may not be aware of, which will allow us to think of the question we ask or the test we perform in a more objective way, hopefully reducing the uncertainty in our decision-making process along the way.

Thomas Bayes, an English clergyman and statistician, is credited with the theorem that bears his name. In terms useful to our discussion, Bayes' theorem provides a formula for calculating the probability of the presence of disease after eliciting some information in the history or receiving a positive or negative test result. This can be demonstrated through our D-dimer case described above, but first, we need to familiarize ourselves with a few formulas.

The odds of a disease being present refer to the number of times it occurs divided by the number of times it does not occur. Or, in formula terms:

$$\text{Odds} = \text{probability}/ (1 - \text{probability}) \text{ or } O = P/(1 - P)$$

The probability of a disease, on the other hand, refers to the number of times it occurs divided by the number of times it could occur, or

$$\text{Probability} = \text{odds}/ (1 + \text{odds}) \text{ or } P = O/(1 + O)$$

Another statistical concept important to our discussion here is that of likelihood ratios (LRs). LRs are a different way of measuring diagnostic accuracy when compared with the methods discussed in the previous case. LR can be defined as the ratio of the probability of a particular test result (positive or negative) in those with the disease to the probability in those who do not have the disease. LR can either be

- >1, indicating that the test result is associated with disease presence
- =1, indicating that the test result probability is the same in the presence and absence of disease
- <1, indicating that the test result is associated with disease absence

To help visualize how LRs can be calculated, we will employ one of the examples used in the previous case.

	Disease positive	Disease negative
Test positive	540 (TP)	20 (FP)
Test negative	60 (FN)	380 (TN)

Since a test result may be positive or negative, the LR may be positive (LR +ve) or negative (LR −ve).

The LR +ve is a ratio of the probability of a positive test in the presence of disease (which is the sensitivity of the test) to the probability of a positive test in the absence of disease (which is 1 − specificity):

$$\text{LR +ve} = \text{sensitivity}/ (1 - \text{specificity}) = 0.9/1 - 0.95 = 0.9/0.05 = 18$$

In this case, a positive test is 18 times more likely in the presence of disease than in the absence of disease (effectively nailing the presence of disease in this patient).

The LR −ve is a ratio of the probability of a negative test in the presence of disease (which is 1 − sensitivity) to the probability of a negative test in the absence of disease (which is the specificity):

$$\text{LR −ve} = (1 - \text{sensitivity})/\text{specificity} = 1 - 0.9/0.95 = 0.1/0.95 = 0.1$$

This indicates a 10-fold decrease in the odds of having the disease when the result is negative (virtually ruling out any chance that the patient may have the disease).

Having, hopefully, grasped the above concepts regarding probabilities, odds and LRs, we can return our attention to Bayes' theorem. Bayes' theorem will allow us to calculate the post-test probability of a condition using the formula below:

$$\text{Post-test odds} = \text{pre-test odds} \times \text{LR}$$

We can now use the case on which this is based. We will assume that our colleague thought the risk of this patient having a DVT was 5% prior to ordering the D-dimer test. This risk was determined by, one may presume, the lack of risk factors and an unconvincing clinical presentation. The sensitivity of this particular D-dimer assay is 90%, and the specificity is 50%. Bayes' theorem is deployed as follows:

$$\text{Pre-test probability} = 5\% = 0.05$$

$$\text{Pre-test odds} = P/1 - P = 0.05/(1 - 0.05) = 0.052$$

In this case, the patient had a positive D-dimer result, so we will use the LR +ve formula:

$$\text{LR +ve} = 0.90/(1 - 0.50) = 1.8$$

$$\text{Post-test odds} = 0.052 \times 1.8 = 0.0936$$

$$\text{Post-test probability} = O/1 + O = 0.0936/(1 + 0.0936) = 0.085$$

So, after a positive test, the probability of a DVT in this patient is 8.5%. The test, therefore, has only increased the probability of the diagnosis by 3.5% (from a pre-test probability of 5% to a post-test probability of 8.5%). Has the positive test really changed the possible likelihood of the presence of a DVT? Was it a test worth doing, or would it have been more prudent to organize further investigations at the time of the original presentation? This would certainly make an interesting discussion between the on-call doctor and their colleague who ordered the test.

Let us see how a negative test result could have altered the discussion:

$$\text{Pre-test probability} = 0.05$$

$$\text{Pre-test odds} = 0.05/(1 - 0.05) = 0.052$$

$$\text{LR} -ve = (1 - 0.9)/0.5 = 0.2$$

$$\text{Post-test odds} = 0.052 \times 0.2 = 0.010$$

$$\text{Post-test probability} = 0.010/(1 + 0.010) = 0.009$$

A negative test result would have reduced the probability of a DVT in this patient to 0.9%, which would have effectively ruled out the disease. This would have saved the patient from potentially more invasive testing and wasted time at the hospital: a case that the colleague may be keen to make.

So, how can one apply Bayes' theorem to one's practice in a more practical way? The concepts of Bayes' theorem could be applied in a qualitative way (Medow, 2011). The pre-test probability can be classified as varying from very unlikely to very likely. One could argue that if a disease is either very unlikely or very likely, there is hardly any benefit in carrying out a test, as it will either confirm what is already highly suspected or not shift the post-test probability sufficiently enough to rule out or rule in the disease. Trainees and trainers can discuss the following scenarios and determine the best course of action based on Bayes' theorem (would the proposed intervention sufficiently alter the likelihood of disease?).

1. A 75-year-old smoker calls and informs you he is getting central chest pain, which has been intermittently present for the last six hours. It is occasionally worse with exertion but has been present at rest as well. He has felt slightly short of breath with it, but this has not been persistent. He is currently on amlodipine for hypertension. Would you call the patient in for an electrocardiogram (ECG) or ask the patient to attend casualty for serial ECGs and a troponin blood test?

2. A 44-year-old man calls about a sudden onset of a headache three hours ago; akin to being hit with a bat at the back of the head. The initial headache was intense in nature, and he vomited once. Since he has suffered from migraines in the past, he took his usual migraine medication and tried to sleep the headache off. He says the headache has eased slightly but still remains in the background, and although he has not vomited again, he remains nauseous. Should the patient be called in for a neurological examination, or should he attend casualty for imaging of his brain?

After discussion, one may conclude that there are certain conditions that are serious enough to warrant further investigations to definitively rule them either in or out, even when the clinician may think that they are unlikely. As a rule, one can refer back to the triad of hypervigilance (Figure 1.2 on page 6); if a condition fits the criteria, then a patient would be better served by a more definitive investigation rather than an intervention (single ECG, neurological examination or D-dimer) that will serve little to reassure the patient and the clinician.

Learning Tip

We established in the previous case that statistics are our friend in managing medical certainty. However, one must not rely on them solely. As Mark Twain once remarked, "Facts are stubborn, but statistics are more pliable"; we must have other mechanisms in place to deal with the inevitable uncertainty that is the hallmark of clinical practice. Appropriate safety netting, arranging follow-up, discussing with colleagues and enhancing one's knowledge around the subject by constant reading and reflection are important tools for the safe practice of medicine.

AKT PREPARATION

Options for questions 46–50:

a. 10%
b. 10
c. 20%
d. 20
e. 1
f. 0.1%
g. 100%
h. 1000
i. 50

Questions 46–50 refer to the scenario regarding a recent study mentioned below. For questions 46–50, pick the correct answer from the options above.

A representative of a drug company attends your surgery to tell you about a new drug, X, on the market. It has shown promising results in the treatment of disease Q, and the drug company feels that it should be considered for prescribing in all eligible patients. In a recent trial, 200,000 patients were recruited. There were 100,000 patients in the control arm and another 100,000 in the treatment arm. After one year of treatment with drug X, 400 patients developed disease Q. In the control arm, which included patients with no treatment, 500 patients developed the disease.

46. What is the relative risk reduction (RRR) associated with drug X?

47. What is the absolute risk reduction (ARR) in the treatment arm?

48. What is the number needed to treat (NNT)?

49. Consider the same drug X being used to treat a rarer condition Y. In this trial, 250 patients in the control arm of 100,000 developed condition Y. The drug company still reports a 20% RRR in the treatment arm. Which of the following statements is/ are true?

  a. The absolute risk reduction (ARR) is likely to be greater as the condition is rarer.
  b. The NNT will be less than 1000.
  c. The NNT will be greater than 1000.
  d. The NNT is not affected as the RRR is the same.
  e. None of the above.

50. You receive a letter from your local public health department informing you of an *E. coli* outbreak amongst staff at the local hospital. Food served in the staff canteen is considered a likely source. Figures show that there are 45 affected staff members, 35 of whom ate at the staff canteen. For the purposes of investigation, a control group of 180 staff members who did not develop *E. coli* was used. Of these 180 staff members, 60 had eaten at the staff canteen. Which of the following statements is false?

  a. This is an example of a case–control study.
  b. An odds ratio greater than 1 proves that exposure causes the outcome being studied.
  c. Odds ratio calculation can be used to study the relationship between exposure and outcome.
  d. An odds ratio of 1 implies that exposure does not affect the odds of the outcome.
  e. An odds ratio of less than 1 suggests exposure is associated with reduced odds of the outcome.

BIBLIOGRAPHY

Deeks JJ, Altman DG. Diagnostic tests 4: Likelihood ratios. *BMJ* 2004 Jul 17; **329**(7458): 168–9.
Duffett L, Castellucci LA, Forgie MA. Pulmonary embolism: Update on management and controversies. *BMJ* 2020; **370**:m2177.
Medow MA, Lucey CR. A qualitative approach to Bayes' theorem. *BMJ Evid Based Med* 2011; **16**:163–7.
Meyer AND, Giardina TD, Khawaja L, Singh H. Patient and clinician experiences of uncertainty in the diagnostic process: Current understanding and future directions. *Patient Educ Couns* 2021 Nov; **104**(11):2606–15.
Szumilas M. Explaining odds ratios. *J Can Acad Child Adolesc Psychiatry* 2010 Aug; **19**(3): 227–9.

11

Case 11: Recurrent abdominal pain

An eight-year-old child is back in your clinic again with her third episode of abdominal pain in three months. Since the previous night, she has been getting griping central abdominal pains associated with flatulence and repeated visits to the toilet. Defecation seems to ease the pain for a short period, but then the pain returns again. She describes her stool as a little loose but denies diarrhoea. She has no fever, and the pain is similar in nature to the episode she had the previous month. She (and the rest of the family) has been up all night with it. You note that she went through a similar phase six months ago, when she would frequently attend the surgery with similar symptoms. All investigations (full blood count, renal and liver function, erythrocyte sedimentation rate, coeliac screen, and urine and stool microscopy) had been normal, and the child had continued to gain weight at a satisfactory rate. Mum would like her to be referred for a "scan" as "something must be wrong". These recurring episodes are impacting her attendance at school and causing a lot of stress at home too.

Which of the following statement(s) is/are true?

a. An ultrasound scan of the abdomen is unlikely to yield a positive result in this case.
b. The underlying cause of her pain is likely to be a complicated interplay between biological, social and psychological factors.
c. Original studies by John Apley looking into recurrent abdominal pain (RAP) of childhood estimated an underlying organic cause in 30% of children.
d. The child should be prescribed a trial of pizotifen, as there is evidence of its benefit in such cases of abdominal pain.
e. An increasing body of evidence supports the withdrawal of lactose from the diet to help with recurring abdominal pain.

DOI: 10.1201/9781003449737-12

ANSWER

a and b are true

Recurrent abdominal pain was first described in 1958 by John Apley. In this landmark study, which looked at 1000 children at primary and secondary schools in Bristol (hence, making it very relevant to general practice), recurrent abdominal pain was defined as at least three bouts of abdominal pain, severe enough to cause functional impairment in the child, over a period of three months. The purpose of the study was to identify the type of children who get abdominal pain. Although conducted over 50 years ago, the study remains an interesting and remarkably valid review of the problem. The study showed a slightly increased prevalence amongst girls (12.3% vs 9.5%) with a peak occurring (in girls) between the ages of eight and ten. Apley found the children who suffered from RAP were more likely to be "highly-strung, fussy, excitable, anxious, timid and apprehensive". He also observed that they were more likely to have undue fears, suffer from nocturnal enuresis and sleep disorders, and have appetite difficulties. Approaching the matter holistically, Apley was keen to determine a profile of the family of the child suffering from RAP. He found that parents and siblings of children who suffer from RAP were more likely to have suffered from RAP themselves. In the majority of these cases, the family member would be the mother. Other common family complaints were migraines, history of peptic ulcer and "nervous breakdowns". The majority of the children complained of pain in and around the umbilicus. Other reported associated disturbances were pallor, vomiting, fever, headache and subsequent sleepiness or lethargy.

Fifty years on, and RAP remains a challenging condition to manage. The first step in dealing with RAP is to rule out an underlying organic problem. Primary care physicians now have access to a greater number of investigations than Apley did 50 years ago. This allows a more complete assessment of the problem but also, unfortunately, may identify minor, insignificant problems, which can result in unnecessary anxiety and treatment for the child. Organic disease is thought to account for 5–10% of cases of RAP in the community. However, other studies, particularly those carried out on children referred to secondary care, have found organic pathology to be much more common. El-Matary et al. looked at 103 children with RAP and found that organic disease accounted for a third of cases. Apart from a detailed questionnaire and full physical examination, all children were screened for coeliac disease and *Helicobacter pylori* infection and had a full blood count, inflammatory markers, serum amylase, liver function test, stool and urine analysis, and an abdominal ultrasound performed. A history suggestive of gastroesophageal reflux disease (GERD) resulted in endoscopy and oesophageal pH monitoring. A history of abdominal pain at night and abdominal tenderness on clinical examination was more likely to be associated with an organic underlying cause. Like Apley, they found abdominal pain that was centred around the umbilicus was less likely to be due to an organic cause. Some of the more organic causes identified in various studies include *Helicobacter pylori* infection, a slow transit gut, urinary tract infections and disorders, constipation, GERD, coeliac disease and food intolerance. Stool, urine and serum analysis (with the addition of serum glucose measurement to the list above) is not an unreasonable set of initial investigations. Further investigations and referral to secondary care will generally depend upon the results, the course of abdominal pain after initial reassurance and the extent of parental concern.

> ### Learning Tip
>
> Identifying and evaluating red flags is an integral part of primary care practice. They serve as markers for increased suspicion in a whole variety of clinical presentations such as headache, back pain, red eye and dyspepsia. Their presence should trigger off further investigation and referral as appropriate. This minimizes the risk of missing serious conditions in primary care. Red flags for recurrent abdominal pain in children include fever, pain located away from the periumbilical area, tenderness on examination, raised erythrocyte sedimentation rate (ESR), weight loss and stunting of growth.

The Rome IV Diagnostic Criteria for Disorders of Gut–Brain Interaction (DGBI) aims to classify functional abdominal pain (no organic cause) in children in order to assist diagnosis and management. It subdivides functional abdominal pain in children into four separate categories. Each category has its own diagnostic criteria in terms of nature and duration of symptom presence:

1. Functional dyspepsia
2. Irritable bowel syndrome
3. Abdominal migraine
4. Functional abdominal pain-not-otherwise specified

It is debatable whether applying strict diagnostic criteria to functional disorders in children leads to better treatment strategies and improved outcomes, but the classification does allow some structure to the management when approaching this problem in a clinical setting.

The mainstay of management in RAP is reassurance. Many parents and children are reassured by an explanation and a normal set of initial investigations. Therapeutic options may be classified as pharmacological, psychosocial and dietary. The success of pharmacological therapy may be determined by the underlying cause of the pain. Simple analgesics may be used during flare-ups. Parents should be advised not give analgesia "prophylactically", as RAP is a fluctuating condition and natural pain-free days should not be attributed to the analgesic drugs. The serotonin antagonist pizotifen has been shown to be effective in the prophylaxis of abdominal migraine. Symon et al. looked at 16 children between the ages of 5 and 13, and found that children receiving pizotifen had fewer days of abdominal pain. Two children reported side effects: drowsiness and weight gain. Another trial (See et al.) reported a subjective benefit in children with RAP and dyspepsia when treated with the H2-receptor antagonist famotidine compared with placebo. Only 25 children were included in this study. Kline et al. reported a benefit in 75% of the 42 children recruited in their study when treated with peppermint oil for irritable bowel syndrome (IBS). However, a Cochrane review looking at 16 studies concluded that there was insufficient evidence supporting the use of drugs in the management of RAP (Martin et al., 2017).

A more helpful approach would be to consider RAP in the context of a biopsychosocial model of disease. Although there may be underlying biological mechanisms responsible for the symptoms (e.g., visceral hyperalgesia, gut dysmotility or autonomic nervous system instability), it is more likely that they are a manifestation of a complex interplay between underlying biology, the child's psychological make-up, and social interactions within the family and school environment. As a result, psychological interventions such as cognitive behavioural therapy and family therapy have been tried with some success in RAP. Access to such interventions is generally limited, making it difficult for them to be routinely used.

Despite the lack of good-quality evidence in favour of suggesting diet modification, it remains a commonly used strategy in RAP. Children participating in Apley's original study were specifically asked about their milk drinking habits, as it was felt that excessive consumption might be linked with RAP. Apley found that children who suffered from RAP tended to drink less milk than controls. Subsequent studies (Lebenthal, Dearlove) have looked at lactose avoidance as a possible management strategy but failed to show a benefit. Based on this, a prolonged trial of lactose-free diet cannot be advised, but a short trial may be considered along with other management techniques. An increase in fibre intake may also be suggested, despite unreliable and inconclusive data from clinical studies. Gawronska et al. looked at dietary supplementation with Lactobacillus in 104 children. Children were classified according to Rome II criteria as having either irritable bowel syndrome (IBS), functional dyspepsia or functional abdominal pain. Children with IBS receiving Lactobacillus were more likely to have fewer episodes of pain when compared with those receiving placebo (it did not, however, reduce severity of pain). No differences were found in the functional dyspepsia or functional abdominal pain groups. Success with a single dietary component is unlikely, and management should involve getting the child to keep a food and pain diary. Suggestions of additions or avoidance of certain foods can then be based on the information derived from such charts.

AKT PREPARATION

Options for questions 51–55:

a. Intussusception
b. Acute appendicitis
c. Pyloric stenosis
d. Haematocolpos
e. Testicular torsion
f. Strangulated inguinal hernia
g. Idiopathic scrotal oedema
h. Wilkie's syndrome
i. Infantile colic

Questions 51–55 refer to children presenting with abdominal pain. Choose the most appropriate answer from the list above. Each option may be used once, more than once or not at all.

51. A 15-year-old girl, with normal development of secondary sexual characteristics, presents with amenorrhoea, cyclical abdominal pain and the presence of an abdominal mass.

52. A six-month-old boy presents with intense crying, drawing up of knees, sporadic vomiting and redcurrant jelly stools. Mum tells you she started weaning him three days ago.

53. Hypochloraemic alkalosis is discovered in a four-week-old girl presenting with worsening vomiting.

54. Which of the following statements regarding male infant circumcision are true?

   a. Male circumcision is associated with a protective effect against the acquisition of HIV in heterosexual males in areas of high HIV prevalence.
   b. There is strong evidence that male circumcision is associated with a reduced risk of developing gonorrhoea and Chlamydia.
   c. Circumcision appears to be protective against the development of a urinary tract infection (UTI) in boys under the age of two.
   d. Male circumcision is associated with a lower risk of invasive penile cancer but a slightly increased risk of cervical cancer in the female partner.
   e. Male infant circumcision is associated with reduced sexual satisfaction and sexual function compared with non-circumcised men.

55. Which of the following tumours is associated with aniridia?

   a. Neuroblastoma
   b. Wilms' tumour
   c. Non-Hodgkin's lymphoma
   d. Rhabdomyosarcoma
   e. Ewing's sarcoma

BIBLIOGRAPHY

American Academy of Pediatrics Task Force on Circumcision. Male circumcision. *Pediatrics* 2012 Sep; **130**(3):e756–85.

Apley J, Naish N. Recurrent abdominal pains: A field survey of 1,000 school children. *Arch Dis Child* 1958; **33**(168):165–70.

Ceccuti A. Case report: Haematocolpos with imperforate hymen. *Can Med Assoc J* 1964; **90**(25):1420–1.

Davidoff AM. Wilms tumor. *Adv Pediatr* 2012; **59**(1):247–67. doi: 10.1016/j. yapd.2012.04.001

Dearlove J, Dearlove B, Pearl K *et al.* Dietary lactose and the child with abdominal pain. *Br Med J (Clin Res Ed)* 1983; **286**(6382):1936.

El-Matary W, Spray C, Sandhu B. Irritable bowel syndrome: The commonest cause of recurrent abdominal pain in children. *Eur J Pediatr* 2004; **163**(10):584–8.

Gawrońska A, Dziechciarz P, Horvath A *et al.* A randomized double-blind placebo-controlled trial of Lactobacillus GG for abdominal pain disorders in children. *Aliment Pharmacol Ther* 2007; **25**(2):177–84.

Huertas-Ceballos A, Logan S, Bennett C *et al.* Psychosocial interventions for recurrent abdominal pain (RAP) and irritable bowel syndrome (IBS) in childhood. *Cochrane Database Syst Rev* 2008 Jan 23;(1):CD003014.

Huertas-Ceballos A, Logan S, Bennett C *et al.* Dietary interventions for recurrent abdominal pain (RAP) and irritable bowel syndrome (IBS) in childhood. *Cochrane Database Syst Rev* 2009 Jan 21;(1):CD003019.

Hulka F, Campbell TJ, Campbell JR *et al.* Evolution in the recognition of infantile hypertrophic pyloric stenosis. *Pediatrics* 1997 Aug; **100**(2):E9.

Kline RM, Kline JJ, Di Palma J *et al.* Enteric-coated, pH-dependent peppermint oil capsules for the treatment of irritable bowel syndrome in children. *J Pediatr* 2001 Jan; **138**(1):125–8.

Lebenthal E, Rossi TM, Nord KS *et al.* Recurrent abdominal pain and lactose absorption in children. *Pediatrics* 1981; **67**(6):828–32.

Liberman M, Daily B. *Paediatrics What Shall I Do?* Butterworth-Heinemann Ltd; 1993.

MacKinlay GA, Watson ACH. Surgical paediatrics. In: Campbell AGM, McIntosh N. *Forfar & Arneil's Textbook of Pediatrics.* Churchill Livingstone; 1998. P. 1768–1801.

Martin AE, Newlove-Delgado TV, Abbott RA *et al.* Pharmacological interventions for recurrent abdominal pain in childhood. *Cochrane Database Syst Rev* 2017; **3**(3):CD010973.

Motamed F, Mohsenipour R, Seifirad S *et al.* Red flags of organic recurrent abdominal pain in children: Study on 100 subjects. *Iran J Pediatr* 2012 Dec; **22**(4):457–62.

Plunkett A, Beattie RM. Recurrent abdominal pain in childhood. *J R Soc Med* 2005; **98**:101–6.

Ramanayake RPJC, Basnayake BMTK. Evaluation of red flags minimizes missing serious diseases in primary care. *J Family Med Prim Care* 2018; **7**(2):315–18.

Razaq S. *Difficult Cases in Primary Care: Women's Health.* Radcliffe Publishing Ltd; 2012.

See MC, Birnbaum AH, Schechter CB *et al.* Double-blind, placebo-controlled trial of famotidine in children with abdominal pain and dyspepsia: Global and quantitative assessment. *Dig Dis Sci* 2001; **46**(5):985–92.

Symon DN, Russell G. Double blind placebo controlled trial of pizotifen syrup in the treatment of abdominal migraine. *Arch Dis Child* 1995; **72**(1):48–50.

Weydert JA, Ball TM, Davis MF. Systematic review of treatments for recurrent abdominal pain. *Pediatrics* 2003; **111**(1):e1–11.

Wheeler R, Malone P. Male circumcision: Risk versus benefit. *Arch Dis Child* 2013; **98**(5):321–2.

12

Case 12: Pregnancy and sexually transmitted infections

A 22-year-old woman presents to you during a busy morning surgery. She seems quite guarded as she tells you that her period is two weeks late and a pregnancy test carried out the day before was positive. You cautiously congratulate her. She tells you that she has been with a new partner for the last three months and is generally happy about the pregnancy. This is her first pregnancy. As you talk to her about the various aspects of a healthy pregnancy, you note that she remains distant. You politely enquire whether there is something else on her mind. "Doctor, I have noticed some spots down below which are very sore." As you examine her, you realize she is suffering from genital herpes. She asks whether they are likely to harm her baby.

Which of the following is true?

a. Reassuring her that this is a self-limiting condition is the appropriate course of action.
b. Advise the patient that a caesarean section is inevitable.
c. Management of this patient will vary depending on whether this is primary or recurrent herpes.
d. Offer her a termination due to the serious morbidity and mortality associated with neonatal herpes.
e. Risk to the baby is the greatest when genital herpes is acquired in the first trimester.

ANSWER

c is true

Genital herpes simplex virus (HSV) disease is on the rise in the UK. It is estimated that one in eight women has genital herpes in the UK. This makes it quite likely that one may come across women with the condition who are pregnant. Genital herpes is not only a source of great distress to the woman but can have devastating effects on the newborn infant in the form of neonatal HSV infection. This can be caused by either HSV-1 or HSV-2. HSV-1 infection is being increasingly recognized as a cause of genital herpes in the younger population and may be more transmissible to the neonate when compared with HSV-2. The large majority of neonatal infections will result from neonatal exposure to the virus in genital tract secretions during delivery. In utero transmission is considered to be very rare and may occur as a result of infection spreading transplacentally.

The first thing to ascertain is whether this is a case of primary or recurrent genital herpes. This may not be as easy as it sounds. In some cases, the woman will give a clear history of genital herpes in the past, which may be corroborated with her notes confirming this. On the other hand, a previous infection may have been ignored or gone unnoticed due to non-specific symptoms. Studies have also shown than many primary cases of herpes infection are commonly misdiagnosed by clinicians. It is not possible to distinguish between a primary or recurrent infection on clinical examination alone. The reason why the differentiation is so important is that primary infection, particularly acquired in the third trimester, carries the highest risk of transmission to the child causing neonatal herpes. Recurrent herpes in the mother is likely to have resulted in the development of maternal neutralizing antibodies, hence reducing the risk of infection in the infant. For this reason, the diagnosis of suspected genital herpes should be confirmed by swabs taken from the base of the ulcer. If the lesion is vesicular, then it should be de-roofed and a swab of the fluid taken. This will normally require referral to a genitourinary specialist, who may subsequently confirm the diagnosis by viral culture or HSV DNA detection via real time polymerase chain reaction depending on local guidelines and facilities available. The latter method has higher HSV detection rates. HSV antibody testing (IgG to HSV-1 or HSV-2) can also be carried out, which can help determine whether the infection is a recurrent infection. Interpreting these test results, though, is likely to need virology input.

Women with a history of recurrent genital herpes can be reassured that the risk of neonatal transmission and herpes infection is very low. There is also no evidence that their condition will be made worse by pregnancy. Such women should be counselled towards a vaginal delivery. There is a difference of opinion as to how such women should be managed should they develop HSV lesions at the onset of labour. Recurrent genital herpes with active lesions at the onset of labour is associated with a small risk (0–3%) to the baby of neonatal herpes were it to be delivered vaginally. This needs to be offset against the risk of caesarean section to the mother. Despite this low risk to the baby, most mothers in the USA are recommended to have a caesarean section, advice probably influenced by the medico-legal risk. There is evidence that 400 mg of acyclovir taken three times a day in the last four weeks of pregnancy is beneficial, as it reduces the risk of developing a recurrence of HSV at delivery and the chance of a caesarean section being performed. Whether prophylactic antiviral treatment reduces the risk of neonatal HSV infection is unclear.

A woman presenting in pregnancy with primary genital herpes will need to be referred to a specialist genitourinary clinic for the investigations described above. The patient should be screened for other sexually transmitted infections, in particular for HIV, as co-infection results in increased replication of both viruses. She should be treated with acyclovir, oral or intravenous, depending on her clinical condition. Although there is no evidence of teratogenicity, acyclovir is unlicensed in pregnancy. If the presentation is in the first or second trimester, the pregnancy should be managed expectantly with the hope of delivering vaginally at birth. She may also be treated with prophylactic acyclovir from 36 weeks onwards to reduce the risk of developing genital lesions at delivery, although the evidence of benefit of this is lacking. All women developing primary genital HSV in the third trimester should be referred to an obstetrician to discuss operative delivery due to the high risk of neonatal transmission. The risk of transmission is at its highest if the episode of primary infection occurs in the last six weeks of pregnancy. Invasive procedures should be avoided if the woman chooses to have a vaginal delivery. Either way, a neonatologist should be informed of the birth to assess the child, take appropriate swabs and samples, and decide on the need for starting antiviral treatment.

Learning Tip

Recognizing and responding to cues is an important part of the consultation in primary care and therefore an important skill for GP trainees to learn. A cue can be verbal or non-verbal in the form of body language and demeanour. Studies have shown that doctors often fail to pick up on cues. Various reasons could be time pressures, lacking confidence in ability to fix problems that may be perceived as emotional, or simply not noticing them. The last phenomenon is termed "inattentional blindness" by psychologists; the doctor may be so engrossed in solving the task at hand that they may completely lose sight of something else (such as a cue) that is just as important (see Brunet et al., 2021 for more on this).

AKT PREPARATION

Options for questions 56–60:

a. Metronidazole 2 g single dose
b. Benzathine penicillin G 2.4 MU intramuscularly
c. Doxycycline 100 mg twice a day for seven days
d. Lamivudine 100 mg daily
e. Options (c) and (h) combined
f. Acyclovir 800 mg five times a day for seven days
g. Options (a) and (c) combined
h. Ceftriaxone 1 g intramuscularly
i. Cefixime 400 mg orally

Questions 56–60 refer to women presenting with sexually transmitted infections. From the list above, choose the most appropriate (first-line) treatment in each scenario. Each option may be used once, more than once or not at all.

56. A 30-year-old woman develops a painless ulcer on her vulva. Examination of fluid from the ulcer confirms syphilis.

57. A 26-year-old woman presents with dysuria and a mild vaginal discharge. An endocervical swab confirms gonorrhoea.

58. An 18-year-old university student requests contraception on a routine visit. An opportunistic chlamydia screen is positive.

59. Regarding neonatal herpes infection, which of the following statements are true?

   a. Postnatal transmission of virus to the neonate may occur from orolabial lesions.
   b. The highest fatality rate with neonatal herpes is associated with cutaneous disease, which accounts for 45% of clinical manifestations.
   c. Intravenous acyclovir has been shown to reduce mortality when given to infants with central nervous system (CNS) and disseminated disease.
   d. High doses of acyclovir are associated with transient neutropenia in the treated infant.
   e. Cutaneous HSV infection in the newborn responds well to topical acyclovir.

60. Regarding HIV in pregnancy, which of the following statements is/are true?

    a. Breastfeeding is associated with a twofold increase in the rate of HIV transmission.

    b. All pregnant women should be offered screening for HIV at 36 weeks because all transmission from mother to child occurs after this.

    c. In mothers who have HIV and are not taking antiretroviral therapy with a detectable viral load, elective caesarean section is of clear benefit in reducing vertical transmission.

    d. Mothers with HIV should be encouraged to breastfeed early in order to boost the child's immune system against HIV.

    e. A negative HIV antibody test at 18 months confirms that the child is unaffected.

BIBLIOGRAPHY

BASHH and RCOG. *Management of Genital Herpes in Pregnancy.* British Association for Sexual Health and HIV and the Royal College of Obstetricians and Gynaecologists; 2014.

Brunet M, Parkin C, Seeing but not perceiving – Inattentional blindness as a cause of missed cues in the general practice (GP) consultation. *AJPP* 2021; **2**:2–14.

Corey L, Wald A. Maternal and neonatal herpes simplex virus infections. *N Engl J Med* 2009 Oct 1; **361**:1376–85.

Fifer H, Saunders J, Soni S *et al.* UK national guideline for the management of infection with *Neisseria gonorrhoeae. Int J STD AIDS* 2018/2020; **31**(1):4–15.

Foley E. Herpes in pregnancy: How to avoid neonatal transmission. *Br J Sex Med* 2010; **33**(2):4–7.

Hollier LM, Wendel GD. Third trimester antiviral prophylaxis for preventing maternal genital herpes simplex virus (HSV) recurrences and neonatal infection. *Cochrane Database Syst Rev* 2008 Jan **23**;(1):CD004946.

Kingston M, French P, Higgins S *et al.* UK national guidelines on the management of syphilis 2015. *Int J STD AIDS* 2016 May; **27**(6):421–46.

Lazaro N. Sexually transmitted infection in primary care. 2013 (RCGP/BASHH). www.bashh.org/guidelines (Accessed on 15 January 2023).

Nwokolo NC, Dragovic B, Patel S *et al.* UK national guideline for the management of infection with *Chlamydia trachomatis. Int J STD AIDS* 2015/2016 Mar; **27**(4):251–67.

13

Case 13: Parkinson's disease

A 45-year-old male office worker comes to see you. He tells you his older brother has recently been diagnosed with Parkinson's disease (PD) in Australia. As far as he is aware, his parents did not suffer from any neurological illnesses, though his father did develop dementia later on in life. He tells you he has been reading up about the condition and he is concerned that he may also be developing it. He does not have any tremors or gait disorders like his brother, but he has suffered from constipation ever since he can remember, and he has read that this can be an early sign of PD. He would like to discuss with you any tests or treatments on offer that can either confirm the presence of PD or prevent its onset.

Which of the following are recognized as possible prodromal symptoms of PD?

- **a.** Idiopathic REM sleep behaviour disorder
- **b.** Asymmetric vague shoulder pain
- **c.** Hyposmia
- **d.** Depression
- **e.** Cognitive impairment

DOI: 10.1201/9781003449737-14

ANSWER

All of the above are correct

The understanding and management of PD has come a long way since James Parkinson described the "*Shaking Palsy*" almost 200 years ago. In the early part of the 20th century, the demonstration of the loss of dopaminergic neurons in the substantia nigra pars compacta and the presence of Lewy bodies became the anatomical and pathological diagnostic hallmark of PD. Further discoveries about dopamine as a neurotransmitter heralded the introduction of L-3,4-dihydroxyphenylalanine (L-DOPA) as an effective treatment option for PD.

The development of acute parkinsonism in a group of seven unfortunate heroin users in the 1980s led to further breakthroughs in the understanding of the condition. Heroin, contaminated with a toxin called MPTP, resulted in a neurological condition indistinguishable from PD. Once identified as the culprit, MPTP spurred further research into how PD develops in primates injected with MPTP, which shed invaluable light on the pathophysiology of the condition. Later developments in genetic analysis allowed the identification of mutations in the *SNCA* gene, coding for the protein alpha-synuclein (α-syn), which leads to the accumulation of this protein in the formerly identified Lewy bodies. Other genetic mutations linked with PD have since been identified and have formed the basis of potential gene therapies.

The rapid rise in cases of PD worldwide has led to many experts likening it to a pandemic. Epidemiological data suggests that PD is likely to be the fastest-growing neurological condition in the world. It appears that this increase cannot be wholly accounted for by an ageing population or by improved diagnostic skills. This has led researchers to look for environmental causes to help explain this rapid increase in the incidence and prevalence of PD. Environmental pollution and increased use of toxic pesticides and chemicals linked with industrialization have been postulated as underlying reasons for this increase. Reduced smoking due to aggressive campaigns has also been linked with an increase in PD. The gut biome also seems to be emerging as a credible link to the underlying increase in PD cases. Constipation being a common prodromal symptom in PD patients suggests the possibility of gut inflammation and malfunction linked to alterations to the normal gut microbiota.

Despite the advances in the understanding of the condition, the diagnosis of PD remains, primarily, a clinical one. Suspicion of the presence of disease is often raised in primary care. The presence of bradykinesia, a unilateral resting tremor, limb rigidity, shuffling gait, difficulty turning in a single movement, mask-like facial features and micrographia all raise the suspicion of the presence of PD. However, the presence of certain symptoms are considered as "red flags" and should raise the suspicion of atypical parkinsonism or an alternative neurodegenerative disorder. Red flag symptoms include:

- **Early falls**: Although falling in late PD is common, patients presenting with falls early in their presentation could indicate atypical disease. Falling backwards with postural instability should raise the suspicion of progressive supranuclear palsy (PSP).
- **Severe autonomic dysfunction**: Much like falls, PD patients will have a degree of autonomic dysfunction in relation to blood pressure and urinary continence. However, if the autonomic dysfunction is severe and early in presentation, conditions such as multiple system atrophy (MSA) should be considered.
- **Gait abnormalities**: Shuffling gait with difficulty turning is often seen in PD, as discussed above. However, suggestions of cerebellar involvement presenting with ataxia and broad-based gait raises the suspicion of MSA or other neurodegenerative disorders. Axial rigidity and postural instability in PSP can also result in a stiff and clumsy gait, which can often be mistaken for PD.
- **Cognitive impairment**: Fluctuating cognition with vivid visual hallucinations suggests dementia with Lewy bodies but can sometimes be difficult to differentiate from PD dementia.
- **Speech abnormalities**: Severe speech abnormalities with motor dysfunction in a limb ("not doing what it is told to do") suggest the possibility of corticobasal syndrome.

This is not an exhaustive list of symptoms or conditions that can be confused with PD. However, making the exact diagnosis remains the function of the neurologist or geriatrician, and it would suffice the primary care physician to just be wary of alternative presentations of PD-like disorders.

The growing recognition of prodromal symptoms of PD opens up an interesting but challenging avenue for primary care physicians. The non-motor nature of most of the prodromal symptoms goes against the common perception of PD being a motor disorder. The symptoms discussed in the case above are sufficiently common to be present for decades before a formal diagnosis of PD is made. However, once the motor symptoms appear, directly asking the patient regarding the presence of any of the prodromal symptoms can be useful in making the diagnosis. In the scenario above, it is questionable how relevant the presence of constipation is. Moreover, until disease-modifying drugs for PD are developed, their relevance in the management and diagnosis of PD remains limited. There may be select cases where genetic testing may play a role, where prodromal symptoms develop in a patient with a close relative with a specific type of genetic PD. Nonetheless, since current treatments of PD are designed primarily for symptom control rather than disease modification, the presence of any prodromal symptoms is irrelevant until symptoms arise that the patient feels will benefit from treatment. This, however, remains an interesting avenue of research, and online calculators have been developed, which allow a risk of developing PD to be calculated from the presence or absence of various prodromal symptoms that are being researched. Their usefulness to primary care physicians is limited, and they are primarily used by specialists, particularly for the purpose of research. It is a field to be aware of, as future developments in this area could filter down to primary care to help identify at-risk patients early in their disease presentation and perhaps alter the course of their illness with newer medication.

The heterogeneity of PD presentation and its effects on the patient lend it to a highly individualized management approach. It requires active involvement of the patient themselves. How PD affects an individual will help determine the best way to manage the condition and involves input from the multidisciplinary team and any potential carers also. The mainstay of pharmacological treatment is to replace the depleted dopamine in the striatum or increase the levels of endogenous dopamine. Since dopamine cannot cross the blood–brain barrier (BBB), its levels need to be replenished by alternative means. These include:

- **Levodopa** is the precursor to dopamine and can cross the BBB. It is converted to dopamine by the enzyme DOPA decarboxylase. It can be used to help diagnose PD, as a good response is usually indicative of PD. There had been ongoing concerns regarding early initiation of levodopa hastening disease progression and contributing to levodopa toxicity. However, it is now well established that this is not the case, and there is no reason to delay the start of treatment once the motor symptoms of PD become apparent. The dyskinesia and on-off fluctuations are such significant side effects of levodopa that they become part of the spectrum of disability that PD patients must endure as a result of their illness. Other side effects include nausea, vomiting, anxiety and hallucinations.
- **DOPA decarboxylase inhibitors**: Many of the levodopa side effects occur due to the conversion of levodopa to dopamine peripherally, prior to crossing the BBB. DOPA decarboxylase inhibitors such as benserazide and carbidopa do not cross the BBB and hence are used in combination with levodopa to minimalize peripheral conversion of the drug, mitigating some of the side effects and allowing lower doses of the drug to be used.
- **Dopamine agonists**: These drugs bind directly to dopaminergic receptors. They may be considered as a first treatment option in younger patients, as they are better

tolerated in this age group and are less likely to be associated with dyskinesias and motor fluctuations when compared with levodopa. A worrying side effect associated with this class of drugs is the development of impulse control disorder, which can manifest as gambling, hypersexuality and binge eating. Abrupt withdrawal from the drug can induce intense agitation and anxiety and should be avoided under all circumstances. Commonly used drugs in this class include ropinirole, rotigotine, pramipexole and apomorphine.

- **Monoamine oxidase B (MAO-B) inhibitors**: MAO is involved with the breakdown of dopamine, and so inhibitors of the enzyme, such as seligiline and rasigiline, increase dopamine levels by preventing its breakdown. Since they increase levels of endogenous dopamine, they can be used to delay the start of levodopa if so desired in any particular patient.

- **Catechol-O-methyl transferase (COMT) inhibitors**: COMT is another enzyme responsible for the degradation of dopamine levels. Inhibition of the enzyme with drugs such as entacapone can increase the delivery of dopamine to the striatum. They are often used in combination with levodopa. They can help with the "wearing-off" phenomenon associated with levodopa but can unfortunately make dyskinesias worse.

- **Other non-dopaminergic pharmacotherapy**: Options include anticholinergics. They reduce the activity levels of the neurotransmitter acetylcholine and thus help with the rigidity and tremor associated with PD. However, due to a long list of side effects and poor tolerability in the elderly, they are not often used. The antiviral amantadine is another option when the patient may have problematic rigidity and tremor.

- **Device-aided therapies**: These include deep brain stimulation, levodopa-carbidopa intestinal gel infusion and subcutaneous infusion of the dopamine agonist apomorphine. They are a viable option, in conjunction with patient preference, when the motor fluctuations and dyskinesias of PD persist despite optimizing the above-mentioned pharmacotherapies.

AKT PREPARATION

Options for questions 61–65:

- a. Amyotrophic lateral sclerosis
- b. Multiple sclerosis
- c. Lennox–Gastaut syndrome
- d. Tuberous sclerosis
- e. Bell's palsy
- f. Guillain–Barré syndrome
- g. Myasthenia gravis
- h. Kuru
- i. Huntington's disease

Questions 61–65 refer to neurological conditions. From the list, choose the most appropriate diagnosis for the clinical scenarios described below.

61. A 66-year-old man presents with a six-month history of generalized muscle weakness, which is worse with physical activity and seems to improve with rest. His symptoms seem to be worse after his recent inguinal hernia repair surgery.

62. A 35-year-old man presents with fairly sudden weakness of the left side of the face developing over the course of the morning. He recalls a sensation of fullness in the ear preceding the symptoms. Examination reveals partial weakness affecting all the facial muscles only on the left side.

63. A 44-year-old woman presents with gastroenteritis-like symptoms. She is given supportive advice but returns a few days later complaining of bilateral mild sensory changes in both legs. Examination is reassuring, and a blood test is organized. However, two days later, she is admitted into hospital with bilateral, symmetrical flaccid paralysis of her limbs and breathing difficulties.

64. A 47-year-old smoker presents for his diabetic review. His HbA1c has increased from 53 mmol/mol to 61 mmol/mol over the course of the last year. His 10-year risk of developing CVD is 14% using the QRISK3 assessment tool. He is currently on metformin 1 gram twice a day. Which is the single most appropriate next management option?

    a. Replace metformin with GLP receptor agonist.
    b. Add DPP-4 inhibitor after checking liver and kidney function.
    c. Switch metformin to modified-release preparation.
    d. Add an SGLT2 inhibitor.
    e. Encourage a low-carbohydrate or ketogenic diet and review again in one year.

65. A 54-year-old female with chronic heart failure is counselled for SGLT2 inhibitor initiation. She reveals that she has been on a ketogenic diet for the last two weeks to help aid weight loss. Which is the single most appropriate next management option?

    a. She may commence on an SGLT2 inhibitor provided she regularly monitors her urine for the presence of ketones.
    b. Wait for her to complete the ketogenic diet before starting the SGLT2 inhibitor.
    c. Start and continue the SGLT2 inhibitor as long as she remains euglycemic.
    d. Start the SGLT2 inhibitor as long as the patient gradually weans herself off the ketogenic diet.
    e. She should suspend her ketogenic diet until she is stable on an SGLT2 inhibitor, after which she may restart the diet.

BIBLIOGRAPHY

Connolly BS, Lang AE. Pharmacological treatment of Parkinson's disease: A review. *JAMA* 2014; **311**(16):1670–83.

Dorsey ER, Sherer T, Okun MS, Bloem BR. The emerging evidence of the Parkinson pandemic. *J Parkinsons Dis* 2018; **8**(s1):S3–S8.

Heinzel S, Berg D, Gasser T *et al.* Update of the MDS research criteria for prodromal Parkinson's disease. *Mov Disord* 2019; **34**(10):1464–70.

Holland NJ, Bernstein JM. Bell's palsy. *BMJ Clin Evid* 2014 Apr 9;2014:1204.

Mcfarland NR, Hess CW. Recognizing atypical parkinsonisms: "Red flags" and therapeutic approaches. *Semin Neurol* 2017; **37**(2):215–227.

National Institute for Health and Care Excellence (NICE). (2022) Type 2 diabetes in adults: Management. NG28. Available at https://www.nice.org.uk/guidance/ng28 (Accessed on May 2024).

Nonnekes J, Post B, Tetrud JW. MPTP-induced parkinsonism: An historical case series. *Lancet* 2018;**17**(4):300–301.

Pellicano C, Benincasa D, Pisani V *et al.* Prodromal non-motor symptoms of Parkinson's disease. *Neuropsychiatr Dis Treat* 2007; **3**(1):145–52.

Romano S, Savva GM, Bedarf JR *et al.* Meta-analysis of the Parkinson's disease gut microbiome suggests alterations linked to intestinal inflammation. *NPJ Parkinsons Dis* 2021; **7**(1):27.

Roos DS, Klein M, Deeg DJH *et al.* Prevalence of prodromal symptoms of Parkinson's disease in the late middle-aged population. *J Parkinsons Dis* 2022; **12**(3):967–974.

Shahrizaila N, Lehmann HC, Kuwabara S. Guillain-Barré syndrome. *Lancet* 2021 Mar 27; **397**(10280):1214–28.

Somagutta MKR, Uday U, Shama N *et al.* Dietary changes leading to euglycemic diabetic ketoacidosis in sodium-glucose cotransporter-2 inhibitor users: A challenge for primary care physicians? *Korean J Fam Med* 2022 Nov; **43**(6):361–66.

Timpka J, Nitu B, Datieva V *et al.* Device-aided treatment strategies in advanced Parkinson's disease. *Int Rev Neurobiol* 2017; **132**:453–74.

Verschuur CVM, Suwijn SR, Boel JA *et al.* Randomized delayed-start trial of levodopa in Parkinson's disease. *N Engl J Med* 2019; **380**:315–24.

Vincent A, Palace J, Hilton-Jones D. Myasthenia gravis. *Lancet* 2001 Jun 30; **357**(9274):2122–8.

Waller S, Williams L, Morales-Briceno H, Fung VSC. The initial diagnosis and management of Parkinson's disease. *Aust J Gen Pract* 2021; **50**(11):793–800.

14

Case 14: Tiredness all the time

Your heart sinks at the sight of the next patient on your list, a 33-year-old woman who has been in and out of your surgery on numerous occasions. She has seen various colleagues with a multitude of symptoms. She complains of tiredness, non-specific muscle aches and bone pain. She has had a whole host of investigations and had also been seen by the local rheumatologist. The diagnosis of chronic fatigue syndrome had been mentioned. A graded exercise programme with the physiotherapist only yielded minimal benefit. A depression screening questionnaire was suggestive of depression. The patient, however, attributed this to her physical symptoms. Two trials of antidepressants were abandoned due to intolerable side effects. She had tried various analgesics for the pain, all either ineffective or intolerable. As you prepare yourself for a 10-minute compassionate listening exercise, she surprises you by asking whether her vitamin D level has been checked during the course of her investigations. Her beautician had commented on it being a possible cause for her brittle nails. You look through her notes and find that a vitamin D level of 15 nmol/L was reported two years ago.

Which of the following statements regarding vitamin D are true?

a. Vitamin D deficiency is a recognized cause of muscle aches and bone pain.
b. Increased vitamin D has been shown to reduce the risk of falls in the elderly.
c. Very low levels of vitamin D are associated with an increased risk of colon, prostate and breast cancer.
d. Vitamin D deficiency has been linked to an increased incidence of mental health disorders such as schizophrenia and depression.
e. Vitamin D supplementation appears to reduce the risk of children developing type I diabetes.

DOI: 10.1201/9781003449737-15

ANSWER

All of the above are true

It is not uncommon in general practice to have patients that fit the above description. Patients presenting with a multitude of symptoms, which are non-resolving, can easily become "heartsink patients". The term "heartsink" was coined by Dr Tom O'Dowd in a 1988 paper in the *BMJ*. The term refers to patients who evoke a somewhat negative response in the doctor due to their repeated presentation with seemingly unresolvable issues. Every GP will have a few under their care. However, it is important to be wary of relevant information getting buried under a mountain of investigations. In this case, a seemingly innocuous omission may have been responsible for many unnecessary investigations and treatments.

With the disappearance of rickets from the medical landscape, vitamin D is rarely thought of as a cause for medical problems anymore. Increasing light is now being shed on the consequences of vitamin D deficiency. This has shown it to be vital for mental and physical well-being and in the prevention of chronic long-term illnesses. With estimates suggesting a possible 1 billion people deficient in vitamin D worldwide, across all age groups, it would not be wrong to call it the silent epidemic. Vitamin D has a particular importance in women, not only due to the impact it has on their health but also due to its effects in pregnancy and during lactation. The Women's Health Initiative (WHI) study showed that women who were vitamin D deficient had a higher risk of colorectal cancer. In addition to increased risk of wheezing and low birth weight, infants born to mothers who were vitamin D deficient late in pregnancy were found to have reduced bone mineral content later in life. Most experts agree that levels below 50 nmol/L would be considered as having inadequate levels of vitamin D, whilst levels below 25 nmol/L are considered deficient.

Vitamin D plays an important role in bone metabolism. In the absence of vitamin D, the gut is unable to absorb dietary calcium and phosphorus effectively. The resultant decrease in calcium levels triggers an increase in parathyroid hormone (PTH) secretion. PTH stimulates osteoclast activity, which dissolves the collagen matrix of bone, thinning bones in the process and causing osteoporosis. PTH also increases phosphate loss in the urine. Low levels of phosphate and calcium result in defective bone mineralization, leading to osteomalacia. Expansion of the poorly mineralized bone caused by hydration is thought to be the underlying cause of bone pain in vitamin D deficiency. Muscle receptors for vitamin D are thought to play an important part in optimal muscle function, with a deficiency leading to muscle weakness and aches. Hence, the low vitamin D levels that were apparently missed in our "heartsink patient" would explain her long-standing muscle aches and bone pain.

So, how can vitamin D be replaced in our patient, and what is the optimal amount? Vitamin D is obtained from sunlight and diet. Oily fish such as salmon, mackerel and sardines and sundried shiitake mushrooms are good dietary sources of vitamin D. Exposure of the arms and legs to the right type of sunlight at the right time of day for 10 minutes can provide up to 3000 IU of vitamin D3. Most tanning beds are also a good source of vitamin D. If all of the above are not possible or insufficient, then one must resort to supplementation. Supplementation may be with vitamin D2 or D3, differing mainly in the way they are manufactured. Vitamin D3 (cholecalciferol) seems to be more effective than vitamin D2 (ergocalciferol) in maintaining vitamin D levels. This allows lower doses of the former to be used. Preparations of vitamin D3 along with calcium are commonly used in those at risk of deficiency and in the management of osteoporosis. A dose of 1000 IU of vitamin D3 daily for adults is effective for maintaining adequate levels. Severe deficiencies may be corrected by higher doses, such as 50,000 IU of vitamin D2 per week for eight weeks followed by monthly doses. A dose of 100,000 IU of vitamin D3 every three months is also an accepted regime. Pregnant or lactating women should take 1000–2000 IU of vitamin D3 per day. Twice this dose for five months is known to be safe in this group. Since 50,000 IU of vitamin D3 per day for five months has been shown to be safe in adults, one should be reasonably reassured that, unless very high doses are ingested for long periods of time, vitamin D intoxication is unlikely. Similarly, vitamin D intoxication cannot take place through excessive sunlight exposure, as any excess vitamin D produced in this way is destroyed by sunlight.

Learning Tip

Contemplating the term "heartsink", it becomes immediately apparent that it refers to a characteristic of the doctor rather than the patient. The negative reaction is induced in the doctor rather than being an objective trait of the patient. Doctors and trainees alike should spend a moment thinking what it is that triggers this emotion in them. It is more likely that the sentiment of a sinking heart is induced by a lack of time or an insufficient grasp of what actually ails the patient. Being wary of one's own limitations and emotional states is likely to reduce the chances of missing an important nugget of information amongst all the background noise in a difficult consultation.

AKT PREPARATION

Options for questions 66–70:

a. Vitamin A
b. Vitamin B
c. Vitamin C
d. Vitamin D
e. Selenium
f. Copper
g. Zinc
h. Iron
i. Vitamin E

Questions 66–70 refer to vitamins and micronutrients and their relation to pregnancy. Pick an answer from the options above. Each answer may be used once, more than once or not at all.

66. Deficiency has been associated with homocysteinemia and poor pregnancy outcomes.

67. Teratogenic when taken in high doses (>10,000 IU/day) in early pregnancy.

68. Level increases in early pregnancy, possibly linked to increased maternal ceruloplasmin levels.

69. The use of folic acid periconceptually is not associated with a reduced risk of which of the following?

    a. Neural tube defects
    b. Cardiovascular defects
    c. Paediatric leukaemia
    d. Limb defects
    e. Twin births

70. Which of the following statements is/are true?

    a. Vitamin B6 has been associated with a reduced risk of dental decay in pregnant women.
    b. Vitamin C is known to increase the bioavailability of dietary non-haem iron.
    c. Zinc supplementation in pregnancy is associated with a reduced birth weight.
    d. Vitamin C requirements in women who smoke are reduced due to its reduced metabolic turnover.
    e. Vitamin D supplementation in pregnancy has been associated with an increased risk of type I diabetes in childhood.

BIBLIOGRAPHY

Allen LH. Multiple micronutrients in pregnancy and lactation: An overview. *Am J Clin Nutr* 2005 May; **81**(5):1206–12.

Holick MF. Vitamin D deficiency. *NEJM* 2007 Jul; **357**(3):266–281.

Levy T, Blickstein I. Does the use of folic acid increase the risk of twinning? *Int J Fertil Womens Med* 2006; **51**(3):130–5.

Lynch SR, Cook JD. Interaction of vitamin C and iron. *Ann N Y Acad Sci* 1980; **355**:32–44.

Mistry HD, Williams PJ. The importance of antioxidant micronutrients in pregnancy. *Oxid Med Cell Longev* 2011; 841749.

Moscrop A. 'Heartsink' patients in general practice: A defining paper, its impact, and psychodynamic potential. *Br J Gen Pract* 2011 May; **61**(586):346–8.

Mulligan ML, Felton SK, Riek AE, Bernal-Mizrachi C. Implications of vitamin D deficiency in pregnancy and lactation. *AJOG* 2010; **202**(5):429.e1.

O'Dowd TC. Five years of heartsink patients in general practice. *BMJ* 1988 Aug 20–27; **297**(6647):528–30.

Rothman KJ, Moore LL, Singer MR *et al.* Teratogenicity of high vitamin A intake. *N Engl J Med* 1995; **333**:1369–73.

15

Case 15: Chronic insomnia

A 45-year-old man attends for an appointment complaining of ongoing issues with his sleep. He reports that he has never been a good sleeper. You note that he has been pre-scribed a number of different sedatives for short periods over the preceding years. Further questioning reveals that there is no pattern to how his sleep is affected: occasionally he has trouble getting off to sleep, and other times he manages to sleep but wakes continu-ously during the night. There is no obvious mood disorder, and it hasn't had an effect on his working life as a busy accountant thus far. It is, however, beginning to cause some self-reported daytime tiredness and lack of concentration. He would like to be prescribed something that he can take on a regular basis which would help him have a more regular sleep pattern but not affect his ability to function during the day.

Which of the following statements is/are true?

a. The diagnosis of insomnia is predominantly an objective diagnosis requiring the presence of certain predefined characteristics.
b. One may be genetically predisposed to insomnia.
c. Women are more likely to be affected by insomnia than men.
d. Sleep deprivation can cause obesity by lowering the levels of satiety signalling hormones.
e. Although not recommended, alcohol before bed is an effective cure for chronic insomnia.

DOI: 10.1201/9781003449737-16

ANSWER

b, c and d are true

Insomnia is commonly encountered in the primary care setting, as the sole presenting reason or as part of a multitude of symptoms. Insomnia is commonly associated with a variety of psychiatric and medical problems, which makes it a challenging presentation to deal with. Moreover, due to a lack of resources for evidence-based non-pharmacological treatments and a dearth of expert interest within defined medical specialties, the primary management of insomnia takes place predominantly in primary care. It is, therefore, vital that the primary care physician is well equipped to deal with insomnia.

Insomnia is a subjective diagnosis and can include any of the subjective descriptors listed below:

- I don't sleep very well.
- I have difficulty getting off to sleep.
- I wake up often through the night.
- I don't feel rested after a night's sleep.
- I wake up too early in the morning.
- I manage to get off to sleep fine but once awake struggle to fall asleep again.
- My child will not sleep on their own or throws a tantrum at sleep time (children).
- My father gets increasingly agitated as evening approaches (sundowning in dementia).

The International Classification of Sleep Disorders, Third Edition (ICSD-3) and the Diagnostic and Statistical Manual of Mental Disorders, Fifth Edition (DSM-5) attempt to present criteria for the diagnosis of insomnia whilst further subdividing it into acute (symptoms less than a month) and chronic (symptoms more than three months). There are only subtle differences between the two nosologies of diagnosis. In practice, though, a strict criteria-based definition is rarely useful. Patients will present primarily with the effects of a lack of sleep, such as daytime tiredness, lack of ability to carry out important daytime functions, poor memory and concentration, sleeping during the day, and a variety of physical and psychological symptoms such as headaches and low mood. Whether the sleep disturbance occurs on at least three nights of the week (criteria for diagnosis in DSM-5) is of much importance is debatable, especially when faced with a patient experiencing significant effects from their lack of sleep.

Differentiating between primary insomnia and secondary insomnia (insomnia caused by an underlying condition, physical or psychological) can be difficult and at times unhelpful. This is because the insomnia can often persist beyond the improvement of the supposed underlying cause, casting doubt on the extent to which the underlying cause was actually responsible for the insomnia (Zucconi, 2021). However, identifying and treating any underlying cause will still be paramount for the successful treatment of the insomnia.

In many cases, patients will volunteer the information regarding what may be causing the insomnia: need to go the toilet, waking in the early hours worried about something, painful or restlessness in legs at night, adjusting to patterns of shift work, etc. A corroborative history from a partner who sleeps with the patient can also be useful as part of the assessment process. They may describe heavy snoring with periods of apnoea (sleep apnoea) or periodic rhythmic, stereotyped and repetitive limb movements or teeth grinding (sleep-related movement disorders). It is important to look at the medications the patient is taking. The problem may be easily resolvable by getting the patient to take their medications, such as diuretics or steroids, in the earlier part of the day. Alcohol does aid sleep in the early part of the night. However, as the alcohol levels drop during the night, it has a detrimental effect on the quality and quantity of sleep. Chronic alcohol usage is associated with chronic insomnia (Colrain, 2014). In teenagers, it is important to explore the usage of electronic devices. Many teenagers will sleep with their phones or tablet devices next to them. Studies have shown that the blue light-emitting diodes (LEDs) of these devices inhibit the secretion of melatonin, thus delaying sleep (Figueiro, 2016).

Learning Tip

Trainers can test the trainee with multiple variations of the presenting history. Some that can be used are

- Primary insomnia
- Insomnia presenting with an underlying psychiatric or psychological cause
- Insomnia due to inappropriate drug or alcohol use
- Insomnia triggered by electronic devices

Ensure that the trainee has taken a complete history and identified the likely cause of the insomnia.

The trainee needs to familiarize themselves with the various treatment options available.

After identifying and addressing the reversible causes of insomnia, we can switch our attention to treatment modalities available for the lack of sleep: cognitive behavioural therapy for insomnia (CBT-I) and medication. CBT-I is a combination of psychological and behavioural techniques that are usually used together to help aid better sleep. The various modalities of CBT-I are listed in Table 15.1 with a brief description of what each one involves. Despite the fact that CBT-I is the recommended form of treatment according to NICE guidelines, the lack of resources and availability often make it difficult to access. As a result, it is important that primary care physicians familiarize themselves with the core principles of each modality so that they are available to offer some assistance and guidance to the patient whilst they wait for more formal treatment. The patient can also be directed towards online CBT programmes such as Sleepio (also recommended by the National Institute for Health and Care Excellence [NICE] and available for free on the NHS in some areas), which can help the patient take charge of their own sleep and create a tailored treatment plan.

Table 15.1   CBT therapies

Type of therapy	What it involves	Advice to patient
Cognitive restructuring	Modifying dysfunctional sleep-related beliefs and thoughts that perpetuate poor sleep	Identify and challenge anxieties and false expectations surrounding poor sleep and its consequences. Patient may have false ideas of what constitutes good sleep or about the negative effects of the lack of it, which puts them in an increasing "anxiety–lack of sleep–anxiety" vicious cycle
Stimulus control therapy	Behavioural techniques aimed at reinforcing the relationship between the bed and only sleep (sex is allowed)	Go to bed only when ready to sleep, get out of the bed if unable to sleep, no electronic devices or books in bed, get out of bed at same time in the morning
Sleep restriction therapy	Limiting bed time to as close as possible to the actual sleep time	Patient keeps a sleep diary to determine actual amount of time spent sleeping. This is then gradually increased in 30-minute intervals over a few weeks until desired sleep duration is achieved. Caution to be used in patients with conditions that may be exacerbated by sleep deprivation, e.g., bipolar disorder
Relaxation training	Teaching patient ways to relax	May involve various methods such as breathing exercises, progressive muscle relaxation, autogenic training and meditation
Sleep hygiene	Behavioural and environmental adjustments to promote better sleep	Appropriate noise and light level of room, avoiding caffeine, exercising on regular basis, optimal room temperature, avoiding alcohol, etc.

CBT-I has consistently been shown to be the most effective treatment for insomnia. However, medications are often used in its management due to the aforementioned lack of access, the acute nature of the presentation, and occasional reluctance of the patient to engage with time-intensive CBT. The ideal medication used would have a quick onset of action and a short half-life, be non-addictive and have few to no side effects. Finding a solution that fits all of the above is difficult in actual practice. NICE recommends a non-benzodiazepine hypnotic used over the course of three to seven days. The non-benzodiazepine benzodiazepine receptor agonists (BzRAs), such as Zopiclone and Zolpidem (commonly known as Z-drugs), are the drugs of choice according to NICE guidelines. They both have relatively short half-life (5 and 2.5 hours, respectively) and therefore reduce the time to onset of sleep. However, too short a half-life and the patient is likely to be awake earlier than desired. Conversely, too long a half-life and the patient is likely to sleep better through the night but have a hangover effect the next morning. Benzodiazepines are best avoided if possible due to their addictive potential.

NICE guidelines also mention the use of modified-release melatonin at a dose of 2 mg for the over 55 year olds. Melatonin is often used in children with insomnia who have learning disabilities or challenging behaviour issues, but this is done under specialist supervision. Melatonin is a prescription-only drug in the UK but is freely available over the counter in many countries and is considered an effective and safe treatment for jet-lag when used for short periods.

Other options include antidepressants such as amitriptyline (half-life up to 28 hours), doxepin and mirtazapine. These antidepressants produce sedation as a useful side effect and can be utilized particularly when depression is presenting alongside the insomnia. Trazodone (a serotonin receptor antagonist and reuptake inhibitor) is another antidepressant that is a safe and alternative option and may have a useful role in managing insomnia in patients with Alzheimer's dementia (McCleery, 2014). Certain antipsychotics, such as quetiapine and olanzapine, also have a useful sedative effect, which can be utilized in certain cases where such drugs are indicated to treat any accompanying psychological distress.

AKT PREPARATION

Options for questions 71–75:

a. Obstructive sleep apnoea
b. Central sleep apnoea
c. Narcolepsy
d. Kleine–Levin syndrome
e. Circadian rhythm sleep–wake disorder
f. Parasomnia
g. Sleep-related movement disorder
h. Fatal familial insomnia
i. Ondine's curse

Questions 71–75 are related to sleep disorders. For questions 71–75, choose the most appropriate diagnosis from the options above. Each option may be used once, more than once or not at all.

71. Mum reports that her four-year-old son occasionally wakes up in the middle of the night confused and disoriented. He remains in his bed and usually doesn't say anything coherent. This lasts for a few moments, after which he goes back to sleep.

72. A 42-year-old male presents with a three-year history of excessive sleepiness in the day. He often falls asleep at his desk at work. More recently, he has had two episodes of totally losing muscle control and collapsing after a bout of laughter, which has triggered his presentation today.

73. A 75-year-old woman describes poor sleep due to an uncontrollable urge to move her legs when she lies in bed. She describes an unpleasant crawling sensation in her legs, which occasionally affects the arms too.

74. Which of the following statements regarding obstructive sleep apnoea (OSA) is false?

    a. OSA has a higher prevalence amongst men.
    b. Polysomnography in a sleep clinic is required to confirm the diagnosis of OSA.
    c. Partners will often report loud snoring and episodes in which the patient stops breathing.
    d. Patients with OSA are at a higher risk of developing cardiovascular disease.
    e. Continuous positive airway pressure (CPAP) is the most effective treatment for most cases of OSA.

75. Which of the following is not routinely monitored through the night during polysomnography?

    a. Brain wave activity
    b. Temperature
    c. Eye movements
    d. Blood oxygen levels
    e. Chest and abdominal movements

BIBLIOGRAPHY

American Academy of Sleep Medicine. *International Classification of Sleep Disorders*, 3rd edn. American Academy of Sleep Medicine; 2014.

American Psychiatric Association. *Diagnostic and Statistical Manual of Mental Disorders*, 5th edn. American Psychiatric Publishing; 2013.

Belanger L, Savard J, Morin CM. Clinical management of insomnia using cognitive therapy. *Behav Sleep Med* 2006; **4**(3):179–98.

Colrain IM, Nicholas CL, Baker FC. Alcohol and the sleeping brain. *Handb Clin Neurol* 2014; **125**:415–31.

Figueiro MG, Overington D. Self-luminous devices and melatonin suppression in adolescents. *Light Res Techno* 2016; **48**:966–75.

Greer S, Goldstein A, Walker, M. The impact of sleep deprivation on food desire in the human brain. *Nat Commun* 2013; **4**:2259.

Herxheimer A, Petrie KJ. Melatonin for the prevention and treatment of jet lag. *Cochrane Database Syst Rev* 2002; **2**:CD001520.

Insomnia. *NICE Clinical Knowledge Summary (CKS)*. Insomnia; 2022. https://cks.nice.org.uk/topics/insomnia/

Irish LA, Kline CE, Gunn HE *et al.* The role of sleep hygiene in promoting public health: A review of empirical evidence. *Sleep Med Rev* 2015; **22**:23–36.

McCleery J, Cohen DA, Sharpley AL. Pharmacotherapies for sleep disturbances in Alzheimer's disease. *Cochrane Database Syst Rev* 2014 Mar 21; **3**:CD009178.

Morin CM, Benca R. Chronic insomnia. *Lancet* 2012 Mar 24; **379**(9821):1129–41.

Nagandla K, De S. Restless leg syndrome: Pathophysiology and modern management. *PMJ* 2013; **89**:402–41.

Ramdurg S. Kleine–Levin syndrome: Etiology, diagnosis, and treatment. *Ann Indian Acad Neurol* 2010 Oct–Dec; **13**(4):241–6.

Spicuzza L, Caruso D, Di Maria G. Obstructive sleep apnoea syndrome and its management. *Ther Adv Chronic Dis* 2015 Sep; **6**(5):273–85.

Walker M. *Why We Sleep*. Penguin Books; 2018.

Zeng L, Zong Q, Yang Y *et al.* Gender difference in the prevalence of insomnia: A meta-analysis of observational studies. *Front Psychiatry* 2020; **11**:577429.

Zucconi M, Ferri R. Classification of sleep disorders. In: Bassetti C, McNicholas W, Paunio T, Peigneux P. *Sleep Medicine Textbook*, 2nd edn. European Sleep Research Society; 2021. P. 151–66.

Case 16: Vertigo

The partner of a 32-year-old woman calls requesting a home visit. He tells you that she had been complaining of a dizzy feeling for a few hours, which suddenly got worse about an hour ago. She described a spinning sensation, feeling imbalanced and nausea. Now, she is too afraid to move and is lying flat on the ground out of fear of her symptoms worsening if she tries to get up. You note that she is a generally fit and well patient and not taking any regular medication. At the home visit, you find her lying on the floor. She denies a headache or any visual disturbance, and her speech is normal. With the help of her partner, she is able to mobilize to the edge of the bed for you to examine her but vomits during the transfer.

Which of the following can help differentiate between the possible underlying causes of her symptoms?

a. The presence or absence of hearing loss.
b. The presence of a concurrent viral illness.
c. A negative head impulse test.
d. The presence of unidirectional nystagmus.
e. A positive skew test.

DOI: 10.1201/9781003449737-17

ANSWER

All of the above are correct

Dizziness is a common complaint in primary care, but one that presents a significant challenge in terms of diagnosis and management. This is primarily due to the highly subjective nature of the complaint, which could include light-headedness, an unsteady feeling, pre-syncope, vertigo, or even anxiety or a generally weak feeling. Patients, particularly the elderly, may find it difficult to articulate what they actually mean by the term, leaving the physician to try to elucidate what exactly it is that the patient is experiencing. Vertigo is a form of dizziness that can be defined as an illusion of movement: the feeling that one is moving when they are not, or the environment around them is spinning or moving. In the murky uncertainty of dizziness, vertigo may be a diagnostic reprieve for the clinician, as it points to a dysfunction of the vestibular system, allowing a more concrete approach to diagnosis and management.

For the primary care physician, the most important differentiation to make is whether the vertigo is due to a peripheral cause or a central cause, the latter requiring input from secondary care. To help us, a simplified version of the vestibular pathway may be represented as follows (Figure 16.1).

The inner ear is composed of the semicircular canals (detecting angular acceleration of the head) and the otolith organs: the utricle and saccule (detecting linear acceleration and spatial orientation of the head). Afferent nerves from each inner ear carry signals to the vestibular nuclei in the brainstem via the vestibular portion of the vestibulocochlear nerve. The vestibular nuclei have multiple projections connecting them, back and forth, with other pathways important for balance (such as vision and proprioception) and the cerebellum. An asymmetry in this system, anywhere along the peripheral and central pathways, results in vertigo. Due to the incredibly complex connections between the various centres controlling balance and the possibility of the vertigo arising from lesions anywhere along these pathways, it is difficult to give a definitive set of symptoms that are exclusive to either central or peripheral lesions. Differentiation, as always, lies in a careful history and targeted examination to help determine the likely source of the symptoms, resorting to investigations where ambiguity is prevalent.

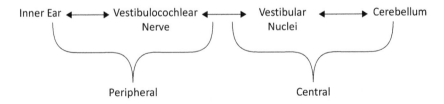

Figure 16.1 The vestibular pathway.

Common peripheral causes of vertigo in primary care include benign paroxysmal positional vertigo (BPPV), labyrinthitis, vestibular neuronitis and Ménière's disease. Central causes include cerebrovascular accident, tumours and multiple sclerosis. The presence of neurological signs and symptoms such as dysarthria, muscle weakness or severe headache will raise the suspicion of a central cause of the vertigo. Although imbalance commonly accompanies vertigo, a complete inability to mobilize or ataxia would also warrant further investigations to rule out a central cause for the vertigo.

A useful technique available to the primary care physician is the HINTS examination. This includes the following examinations:

- Head Impulse
- Nystagmus
- Test of Skew

HEAD IMPULSE

The patient sits facing the examiner. The patient is asked to keep their eyes on the examiner's nose. The head is then turned approximately 20 degrees from the midline and rapidly brought back to the midline. This is repeated on both sides. If, during the movement, the eyes are able to remain fixed on the examiner's nose, then the test is negative and points to a central lesion in the presence of vestibular dysfunction. In a positive test, the eyes will fail to stay fixated on the nose and will move to the midline as the head is brought back to the neutral position. This correction of the eyes is known as a saccade and is indicative of a peripheral lesion being responsible for the vertigo.

NYSTAGMUS

If the vertigo is due to a peripheral lesion, the nystagmus is horizontal or horizontal-torsional and unidirectional. This means that the direction of the nystagmus does not change by changing the direction in which the eyes are fixated. Nystagmus has a slow phase and a fast phase, and its direction is defined by the direction of the fast phase (although it is the direction of the slow phase that localizes the position of the responsible lesion). The nystagmus will also beat faster when the eyes are turned towards the direction of the fast phase of the nystagmus (Alexander's law). Suspect a central cause if the nystagmus is bidirectional (the direction of the fast phase changes as the patient looks left or right) or vertical.

TEST OF SKEW

This test checks for vertical misalignment of the eyes due to a central lesion causing the vertigo. The patient is asked to focus on the examiner's nose again, and one eye is alternatively covered and uncovered. In a positive test, the affected eye will move when covered and then correct itself when uncovered.

The HINTS exam can only have relevance when the vestibular dysfunction is continuous, as in our case above, and not when the symptoms are intermittent. When done correctly, it has been shown to have a sensitivity of 100% and a specificity of 96% for stroke (Kattah, 2009). However, all three components of the HINTS exam need to be present (positive head impulse, unidirectional and horizontal nystagmus, and negative test of skew) to be able to confidently say that the vestibular dysfunction is due to a peripheral lesion.

Learning Tip

The assessment of vertigo can serve as a good clinical case for the trainee. Due to the vast number of conditions that can cause vertigo, it is important that the trainee has a good system for differentiating between the more serious and benign causes of the vestibular dysfunction. This requires targeted history taking and good examination skills, as explained above.

Some of the benign causes, which commonly present in primary care, and their presentation and course are discussed below. The trainee can look up the various causes and then present their system of differentiating between them and their management.

VESTIBULAR NEURITIS (NEURONITIS)

The case at the beginning is likely to represent vestibular neuritis. The damage, as the name suggests, is to the vestibular component of the 8th cranial nerve: the vestibulocochlear nerve. Although the exact cause is unknown, a viral trigger is considered the most likely explanation. Hence, it is often suspected in patients who are suffering or have recently suffered from a viral illness. There seems to be a push to rename this condition acute unilateral peripheral vestibulopathy (AUPVP), as it is unclear whether there is always underlying inflammation of the nerve. The head impulse will be positive (away from the lesion), unidirectional, horizontal or torsional nystagmus may be present, and the test of skew is negative. Symptoms tend to peak over a few days but can persist for weeks afterwards. The patient can be reassured that they do eventually settle with the passage of time.

LABYRINTHITIS

Labyrinthitis has a similar presentation to vestibular neuritis and is caused by inflammation of the labyrinth of the inner ear, most likely secondary to infection. The distinguishing feature from vestibular neuritis is the associated hearing loss, caused by the involvement of the cochlear component of the vestibulocochlear nerve. The sensorineural hearing loss can unfortunately be irreversible. Tinnitus may also accompany the vestibular dysfunction. Although viruses are the commonest cause, bacterial infection of the labyrinth is a possible complication of otitis media.

MÉNIÈRE'S DISEASE

See Case 5.

BENIGN PAROXYSMAL POSITIONAL VERTIGO (BPPV)

BPPV is probably the commonest cause of vertigo in primary care. It is caused by the accumulation of displaced calcium carbonate crystals in the posterior semicircular canal. These misplaced crystals induce hypersensitivity in the semicircular canals to changes in head position. As a result, vertigo is triggered by sudden movements of the head. Nystagmus of a rotational type is usually seen with BPPV. The vertigo and nystagmus are usually of short duration, lasting a few seconds to minutes. The Dix–Hallpike manoeuvre can be used to help diagnose BPPV. The patient sits upright with the head turned approximately 45 degrees in the direction being tested. The patient keeps their eyes open and focuses on a point on a nearby wall. The patient is then made to lie supine quickly with the neck slightly hyperextended. The onset of nystagmus (and possible vertigo and vomiting!) denotes a positive test. If the test is positive, one may proceed from that position to perform the Epley manoeuvre. This is an effective procedure, involving a series of head movements, which is designed to dislodge the errant calcium carbonate crystals from the semicircular canals. Brandt–Daroff exercise can be as effective as the Epley manoeuvre, with the added advantage that it can be carried out at home.

MANAGEMENT

An important principle in the management of vertigo is that in most cases, the intensity of vertigo will dissipate as the triggering factor wanes or compensation occurs. As the brain recognizes an asymmetry between the left and right vestibular organs, it gradually regains balance by the process of compensation. It is therefore advisable to limit the duration of medication use, as its suppressive effect can affect the normal compensatory mechanisms of the brain.

Drug treatment is focused around suppression of the vertigo and the associated nausea and vomiting. Antihistamines such as cinnarizine and promethazine, antiemetics such as metoclopramide, and the phenothiazine prochlorperazine are commonly used as drug treatments for vestibular disorders. Benzodiazepines are also considered effective, particularly for the anxiety induced by the vertigo, but their addictive potential limits their use. Patients suffering from prolonged vertigo or frequent recurrent attacks should be considered for vestibular rehabilitation treatment.

AKT PREPARATION

Options for questions 76–80:

a. Carotid artery stenosis
b. Epilepsy
c. Subclavian steal syndrome
d. Sick sinus syndrome
e. Idiopathic drop attack
f. Postural hypotension
g. Bowhunter's syndrome
h. Micturition syncope
i. Aortic stenosis

Questions 76–80 refer to patients presenting with dizziness. Choose the most appropriate answer from the options above for questions 76–80. Each option may be used once, more than once or not at all.

76. Reception staff press the emergency button after a 48-year-old woman suddenly dropped to the floor whilst waiting in the queue. She did not lose consciousness in the process. She is well known to the practice and has had repeated similar episodes in the last three years. She has been extensively investigated, and no cause has been found.

77. A 54-year-old man presents to the surgery for the third time with vague symptoms of dizziness. Cardiac and neurological examination and blood tests were normal on his previous visits. On this occasion, he has noted that the dizziness is exacerbated by turning his head to the left.

78. A 44-year-old man presents with recurrent bouts of dizziness, blurring of vision, pre-syncope and left arm pain and numbness during exertion. He has been referred to cardiology twice, and no cardiac cause for his symptoms has been found.

79. Which of the following patients is a suitable candidate for the consideration of roflumilast in the management of severe chronic obstructive pulmonary disease (COPD)?

    a. A 76-year-old male on a long-acting muscarinic receptor antagonist (LAMA) with three exacerbations in the last six months.
    b. A 64-year-old female on triple therapy with a history of depression and suicidal ideation having had two exacerbations in the previous 12 months.
    c. A 54-year-old male on a LAMA and long-acting β2-agonist (LABA) recently admitted to the intensive therapy unit (ITU) with a COPD exacerbation.
    d. A 60-year-old female having frequent exacerbations on a LABA and inhaled corticosteroid (ICS) inhaler.
    e. A 70-year-old male with three exacerbations in the previous 12 months who is currently on a LABA/LAMA/ICS combination.

80. A 72-year-old diabetic patient is admitted to hospital with heart failure. Which is the single most appropriate initial medication change that should take place?

   a. Add an SGLT2 inhibitor.
   b. Increase dose of beta-blocker.
   c. Stop pioglitazone.
   d. Add an angiotensin-converting enzyme (ACE) inhibitor.
   e. Add a thiazide diuretic for blood pressure control.

BIBLIOGRAPHY

Baloh RW. Vertigo. *Lancet* 1998; **352**:1841–46.

Cooper CW. Vestibular neuronitis: A review of a common cause of vertigo in general practice. *Br J Gen Pract* 1993; **43**(369):164–7.

Cranfield S, Mackenzie I, Gabbay M. Can GPs diagnose benign paroxysmal positional vertigo and does the Epley manoeuvre work in primary care? *Br J Gen Pract* 2010; **60**(578):698–99.

Dommaraju S, Perera E. An approach to vertigo in general practice. *Aust Fam Physician* 2016; **45**(4):190–4.

Dros J, Maarsingh OR, van der Horst HE *et al.* Tests used to evaluate dizziness in primary care. *CMAJ* 2010; **182**(13):E621–631.

Kattah JC, Talkad AV, Wang DZ *et al.* HINTS to diagnose stroke in the acute vestibular syndrome: Three-step bedside oculomotor examination more sensitive than early MRI diffusion-weighted imaging. *Stroke* 2009; **40**(11):3504–10.

Lacour M, Helmchen C, Vidal P. Vestibular compensation: The neuro-otologist's best friend. *J Neurol* 2016; **263**(Supplement 1):54–64.

Psillas G, Kekes G, Constantinidis J, Triaridis S, Vital V. Subclavian steal syndrome: Neurotological manifestations. *Acta Otorhinolaryngol Ital* 2007 Feb; **27**(1):33–7.

Revell ER, Gillespie D, Morris PG, Stone J. Drop attacks as a subtype of FND: A cognitive behavioural model using grounded theory. *Epilepsy Behav Rep* 2021 Oct 8; **16**:100491.

Roflumilast for treating chronic obstructive pulmonary disease. *Technology Appraisal Guidance* (TA461). 26 July 2017. https://www.nice.org.uk/guidance/ta461

Shahnoor S, Habiba U, Shah HH. Do benzodiazepines have a future in treating acute vertigo? *Ann Med Surg* 2022; **82**:104623.

Taylor WB, Vandergriff CL, Opatowsky MJ, Layton KF. Bowhunter's syndrome diagnosed with provocative digital subtraction cerebral angiography. *Proc (Bayl Univ Med Cent)* 2012 Jan; **25**(1):26–7.

17

Case 17: Polycystic ovarian syndrome

A 22-year-old Asian woman presents to your surgery. She had some blood tests earlier in the week. She tells you she spoke to the receptionist, who told her the bloods had been seen by the doctor, who put a note down saying: "advise appointment with doctor, bloods suggest polycystic ovarian syndrome". She admits being confused, as only two weeks ago she saw your colleague, who told her that her ovaries were normal based on a pelvic ultrasound scan (USS) she had for irregular periods. Looking through her notes, you see that she has been to the surgery on numerous occasions with troublesome acne and facial hair. She has heard of polycystic ovarian syndrome (PCOS), as her Mum was told she suffered from it too. She is keen to get her acne and facial hair sorted, as she is getting married in six months.

Which of the following is NOT amongst the diagnostic criteria for PCOS?

a. 12 or more peripheral follicles on the ovaries
b. Body mass index (BMI) >30
c. Oligo- or anovulation
d. Clinical and/or biochemical signs of hyperandrogenism
e. A raised luteinizing hormone/follicle-stimulating hormone (LH/FSH) ratio

DOI: 10.1201/9781003449737-18

ANSWER

b and e are not amongst the diagnostic criteria of PCOS

Known also as Stein–Leventhal syndrome, after the first researchers to describe the condition in 1935, PCOS is a condition affecting the reproductive, metabolic and cardiovascular well-being of women. Although polycystic ovaries may be seen in up to one in five women, the actual syndrome affects about 6–7% of women in the UK. It is more common amongst women of South Asian origin. Though more common, it is not exclusive to obese women.

This patient's confusion is not entirely misplaced. The medical profession seems to be unclear about the precise definition of the condition also. In 2003, an expert conference in Rotterdam set out to define PCOS and came up with the following recommendation: presence of at least two of the following three would constitute a diagnosis of PCOS, provided other conditions causing irregular periods and hyperandrogenism had been ruled out:

- *Oligo-/anovulation*: This is usually manifested as oligomenorrhoea (fewer than 9 periods in a year or menstrual cycle length greater that 35 days) or amenorrhoea.
- *Evidence of androgen excess*, which may be clinical (acne, hirsutism, male pattern baldness) or biochemical (raised levels of circulating androgens).
- *Polycystic ovaries on USS*.

What is immediately apparent from this definition is that the presence of polycystic ovaries on ultrasound is not necessary for the diagnosis of PCOS. Similarly, the presence of polycystic ovaries on ultrasound does not establish the diagnosis in the absence of other signs and symptoms. This accounts for the quarter of women with normal cycles found to have polycystic ovaries as a coincidental finding on ultrasound. An important point to remember is that a diagnosis of PCOS can only be made when other conditions have been ruled out. These include thyroid disorders, congenital adrenal hyperplasia, hyperprolactinaemia, androgen secreting tumours and Cushing syndrome. Hence, recommended screening tests include thyroid function tests (TFTs), serum prolactin and a free androgen index (FAI).

Although no single underlying aetiological factor is likely to explain all the symptoms and signs of PCOS, there is good evidence that increasing insulin resistance plays a vital role. The resulting increase in insulin production affects the ovaries and the liver separately. In the ovaries, increased insulin (along with higher levels of LH in comparison to FSH) causes thecal hyperplasia, resulting in increased thecal androgen production. In the liver, the increasing levels of insulin reduce the levels of sex hormone binding globulin (SHBG), allowing more testosterone to circulate freely. A large number of the troublesome symptoms of PCOS are caused by the increase in circulating androgens.

It is important that the implications of the condition are discussed with the patient. We will visit each of the consequences of PCOS separately, their possible underlying cause and the various treatments on offer to help the patient.

Menstrual disorders

Irregularities in the menstrual cycle are a common reason for women with PCOS to consult their GP. The rise in circulating androgens arrests the development of follicles, causing anovulation and disruption of the menstrual cycle. Patients should be encouraged to lose weight, as reduction in weight through changes in lifestyle has shown to improve ovulatory function in this group. If regular menstruation is desired, then the oral contraceptive pill may be considered. If contraindicated, cyclical progesterone should be used to induce a withdrawal bleed at least every three to four months. This is because unopposed oestrogen in the premenopausal woman can lead to endometrial hyperplasia and carcinoma. Since increased levels of insulin and increased weight play an important aetiological role in PCOS, treatments to reduce both are being increasingly used in PCOS. Metformin and the thiazolidinediones (TZDs), such as pioglitazone and rosiglitazone, are known to reduce insulin resistance. TZDs, though, are frequently associated with weight gain, perhaps through fluid retention and adipogenesis.

Infertility

Metformin, in particular, seems to be popular amongst gynaecologists, despite its use being unlicensed in PCOS. It is being used to help induce ovulation, particularly in those seeking fertility. There is some evidence that it improves the chances of ovulation, an effect that is enhanced in combination with the antioestrogen drug clomiphene. It may also reduce the risk of miscarriage if taken through pregnancy. Despite the fact that there are no known harmful effects to the growing fetus, metformin is unlicensed for use in pregnancy. TZD use is somewhat stunted due to the concerns of their effect on pregnancy.

Clinical manifestations

Hirsutism and acne are particularly troublesome cutaneous manifestations of PCOS. Treatment involves reducing the amount of circulating androgens and blocking their action at the target site. The combined oral contraceptive pill (COCP) is generally used first line. The oestrogen component of the pill suppresses LH production and also increases the production of SHBG by the liver, thereby reducing the amount of free circulating androgens. The choice of COCP is important, as the progestins vary in their androgenic effects. Drosperinone has antiandrogen activity and hence can be used as part of the COCP (Yasmin). Dianette (ethinylestradiol and the antiandrogen cyproterone acetate) is also licensed for use in the UK. Since metformin improves insulin sensitivity and reduces circulating androgens, it may also be used to treat acne and hirsutism. However, not only is it unlicensed for this indication, but good evidence to support this practice is also lacking. Other licensed treatments for hirsutism include cosmetic measures and topical facial eflornithine. The latter works by inhibiting hair growth and is applied twice daily. A dose of 100–200 mg of spironolactone daily can also be used, though it is unlicensed for this indication. It works by preventing dihydrotestosterone binding to its receptor on the hair follicle.

CARDIOVASCULAR RISK

Women with PCOS are at an increased risk of developing cardiovascular disease. They are also more likely to have impaired glucose tolerance and develop diabetes later in life. Hence, PCOS can be seen as the female version of the metabolic syndrome. An interesting term used to describe this association is "syndrome XX". Insulin resistance in these women, along with a tendency for central adiposity, results in an abnormal increase in free fatty acids, providing the liver substrate for increased triglyceride (TG) production. They also seem to show a higher level of hepatic lipase activity, which increases the conversion of high-density lipoprotein (HDL) to low-density lipoprotein (LDL). The resultant rise in TGs and LDL increases the risk for cardiovascular disease. It should be borne in mind that conventional cardiovascular risk calculators have not been validated in this group. Hypertension should be treated, and a glucose tolerance test should be offered if diabetes is suspected. Obstructive sleep apnoea, an independent risk factor for cardiovascular disease, is also more common in PCOS. If suspected, patients should be referred for nocturnal polysomnography.

Learning Tip

One of the phenomena of modern medicine has been the creation of illness where there was previously none recognized. A patient who does not fulfil the criteria for diabetes may now have pre-diabetes; if the threshold of thyroid-stimulating hormone (TSH) has not been crossed, they have subclinical hypothyroidism; if all the symptoms of coeliac disease are present but the antibody test is negative, we can call it non-coeliac gluten hypersensitivity. "Over-diagnosis" or "over-labelling" brings with it the expectation of treatment, and in many cases, there is no clear consensus on what the treatment should be. In primary care we often find ourselves in these gray areas, diagnosing patients with conditions with no clear diagnostic criteria, let alone recognized evidence-based treatment regimes.

AKT PREPARATION

Options for questions 81–85:

a. Ovarian torsion
b. Dermoid cyst
c. Dysgerminoma
d. Sertoli–Leydig cell tumour
e. Meigs syndrome
f. Premature ovarian failure
g. Ovarian dysgenesis
h. Serous cystadenocarcinoma
i. None of the above

81. A 22-year-old woman presents with amenorrhoea. She complains of hoarseness of voice, troublesome acne and excessive hair. Examination reveals a mass arising from the pelvis and clitoromegaly. USS reveals a unilateral solid ovarian mass.

82. A 70-year-old woman presents with non-specific symptoms of tiredness, cough, shortness of breath and abdominal swelling over the last four weeks. On examination, you find mild ascites and dull percussion note on the right side of chest with reduced air entry. An ultrasound scan reveals an ovarian tumour, which is confirmed as fibroma on histology.

83. A 20-year-old woman presents to the emergency department with severe left-sided abdominal pain for the last one hour. This is associated with nausea and vomiting. Beta human chorionic gonadotropin (B-HCG) and urine dipstick are negative. An ultrasound scan reveals a swollen enlarged left ovary.

84. Which of the following scoring systems may be used for the evaluation of hirsutism in PCOS?

  a. FIGO scoring
  b. Wells score
  c. RMI 1 score
  d. Ferriman–Gallwey score
  e. MASI score

85. Which of the following statements regarding laparoscopic ovarian surgery (LOS) for PCOS is/are true?

  a. Currently, the most widely used surgical technique for ovarian surgery is bilateral wedge resection.
  b. In women who fail to ovulate on clomifene citrate, LOS results in ovulation in about 80% of patients.
  c. LOS is indicated in women who ovulate on clomifene citrate but fail to fall pregnant.
  d. LOS is an effective treatment for acne and hirsutism due to the resulting reduction in circulating androgens following LOS.
  e. Follow-up of women with PCOS post-LOS shows a reduced incidence of cardiovascular disease and diabetes.

BIBLIOGRAPHY

Alam K, Maheshwari V, Rashid S, Bhargava S. Bilateral Sertoli-Leydig cell tumor of the ovary: A rare case report. *Indian J Pathol Microbiol* 2009; **52**:97–9.

Amer SAK. Laparoscopic ovarian surgery for polycystic ovarian syndrome. In: *Recent Advances in Obstetrics and Gynaecology 24*. Edited by Dunlop W, Ledger WL. Royal Society of Medicine Press Ltd; 2008.

Azziz R, Woods KS, Reyna R *et al.* The prevalence and features of the polycystic ovary syndrome in an unselected population. *J Clin Endocrinol Metab* 2004 Jun; **89**(6):2745–9.

Ehrmann AD. Polycystic ovary syndrome. *NEJM* 2005; **352**(12):1223–36.

Fonseca V. Effect of thiazolidinediones on body weight in patients with diabetes mellitus. *Am J Med* 2003; **115**(Suppl 8A):42S–48S. doi:10.1016/j.amjmed.2003.09.005

Gould EA, Kerr HH. Meigs' syndrome: A report of four cases, one having hemohydrothorax. *Ann Surg* 1956; **143**(6):740–3.

Hopkinson ZEC, Sattar N, Fleming R, Greer IA. Polycystic ovarian syndrome: The metabolic syndrome comes to gynaecology. *BMJ* 1998 Aug; **317**:329.

Martin C, Magee K. Case reports: Ovarian torsion in a 20 year old patient. *CJEM* 2006; **8**(2):126–9.

Martin KA, Chang RJ, Ehrmann DA *et al.* Evaluation and treatment of hirsutism in premenopausal women: An endocrine society clinical practice guideline. *J Clin Endocrinol Metab* 2008 Apr; **93**(4):1105–20.

Razaq S. On evidence-based orthodoxy and therapeutic nihilism. *BJGP Life* 2022 Apr 1. https://bjgplife.com/on-evidence-based-orthodoxy-and-therapeutic-nihilism/

Rotterdam ESHRE/ASRM-Sponsored PCOS Consensus Workshop Group. Revised 2003 consensus on diagnostic criteria and long-term health risks related to polycystic ovary syndrome. *Fertil Steril* 2004; **81**(1):19–25.

Royal College of Obstetricians and Gynaecologists. *Long Term Consequences of Polycystic Ovary Syndrome*. Green-Top Guideline No. 33. Royal College of Obstetricians and Gynaecologists; Nov 2014.

18

Case 18: Henoch–Schönlein purpura

The flu season is in full swing, and you have already seen half a dozen kids whom you have diagnosed as having viral upper respiratory tract infections. Next on the list is an eight-year-old boy. He came to see you three days ago with Mum complaining of a runny nose, sore throat and mild cough. Examination had been unremarkable and a viral infection diagnosed. As he settles in the chair, you note that he appears generally well. Mum tells you that he has been complaining of intermittent abdominal pain since yesterday. He vomited twice yesterday but has had no episodes of vomiting today. More worryingly, he has been complaining of pain in his knee joints, which has caused difficulty walking. You examine his abdomen on the couch and note that, though soft on palpation, it is generally tender. As you are examining his knees, a purplish rash over the lateral aspect of his thighs catches your eyes. On closer inspection, this extends over his buttocks and is raised and palpable. You suspect a diagnosis of Henoch–Schönlein purpura (HSP).

Which of the following statements is true?

a. A diagnosis of HSP cannot be made without a lumbar puncture, as bacterial meningitis needs to be excluded as a cause for the purpuric rash.
b. Abdominal pain and arthritis are cardinal features of HSP, occurring in practically all children with the condition.
c. Nine out of 10 cases of HSP will occur in children under the age of 10.
d. IgG is strongly linked with the pathogenesis of the condition, with raised levels almost invariably seen.
e. The multisystem manifestations of HSP rarely settle spontaneously, necessitating steroid treatment in the majority of children.

DOI: 10.1201/9781003449737-19

ANSWER

c is true

HSP derives its name from the descriptions of the condition by Johann Schönlein and his student Eduard Henoch in the 1800s. HSP is a systemic vasculitis of unknown aetiology and is the commonest vasculitic condition of childhood. One study found the estimated annual incidence to be as high as 70.3/100,000 amongst children between the ages of four and seven in the West Midlands (Gardner-Medwin et al., 2002). It is more common in boys. Many infectious pathogens (most commonly group A β-haemolytic streptococcus), immuniza-tions and drugs have been suggested as infectious triggers of the condition, but none have been firmly established as the cause. More recently. it has been linked with influenza vac-cinations during the pandemic of influenza A (H1N1) in 2009 (Watanabe, 2011) and SARS-CoV-2 vaccine and infection (Di Vincenzo et al., 2024). A large majority of cases are in children under the age of 10, but it may occur in adults also, where it may present atypically and in a more severe form. IgA (rather than IgG) is strongly linked with the immunopatho-genesis of the condition, with IgA1 deposits found in the skin, gut and renal mesangium.

In the absence of a specific diagnostic test, diagnosis is based on presenting clinical features. Routine bloods (full blood count, urea, electrolytes and creatinine, clotting screen, liver function tests) and urinalysis should be performed as part of the initial work up on presen-tation. Other tests, such as an autoimmune profile and complement levels, should be per-formed if the diagnosis is in doubt. Since the child with HSP is generally systemically well, a lumbar puncture to exclude bacterial meningitis is not necessary. However, if the diagnosis is unclear or the child is unwell, then other appropriate investigations to determine the source of infection will become necessary. Figure 18.1 lists the important clinical features of HSP.

As the name of the condition suggests, a purpuric rash is the cardinal symptom that allows the diagnosis to be made, as it is present in all cases of HSP. However, it may appear after the onset of other signs and symptoms listed above, making diagnosis of HSP difficult (Mrusek et al.). The rash may initially present as urticaria or erythematous maculopapular lesions progress-ing to a palpable purpura. Oedema and haemorrhage of the bowel, as a result of the vasculitic process, is responsible for the gastrointestinal symptoms. Occasionally, HSP may cause severe abdominal pain, mimicking serious gastrointestinal pathology. Intussusception, perforation and obstruction are rare complications of HSP necessitating further investigations when sus-pected. The arthritis and arthralgia of HSP is particularly debilitating but does not result in last-ing joint damage. Kidney involvement is the most important in terms of long-term sequelae of the condition. Renal manifestations of HSP almost always occur after the onset of the typical purpuric rash. Nephritis will occur in approximately 40% of HSP sufferers (Saulsbury) and will manifest within three months in practically all cases. Hence, GPs should monitor blood pres-sure and urine (in the form of early morning urine dipstick) weekly in the first month of the illness. Thereafter, monitoring can be done fortnightly. If macroscopic haematuria, hyperten-sion or proteinuria is detected, the child should be referred to a paediatrician. These children are likely to need long-term follow-up due to the potential for late deterioration of renal dis-ease (Jauhola et al.). In the absence of the above, less frequent monitoring should be continued.

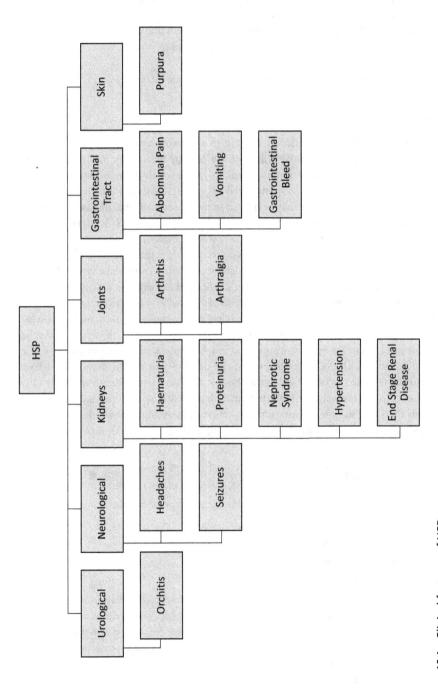

Figure 18.1 Clinical features of HSP.

If blood pressure and urinalysis remain normal a year after the onset of illness, the child and parents can be reassured that the risk of developing renal complications of the illness is very low, and they can be safely discharged from follow-up. If microscopic haematuria persists, yearly urine and blood pressure reviews should continue. Local guidelines may vary on the frequency of reviews needed and should always be referred to.

Treatment of HSP may be considered under two separate categories:

- Rapid relief of symptoms
- Prevention of long-term complications

HSP is a self-limiting condition, recurring in approximately 33% of patients. In the majority of children, the disease will have subsided by four weeks. Bed rest with adequate hydration is generally recommended, as it helps with the resolution of the rash and oedema. Arthritic pain responds well to non-steroidal anti-inflammatory drugs (NSAIDs); however, their use may be limited in the presence of renal disease. Abdominal pain can be distressing and may require opiate analgesia. If this fails, steroids are frequently employed to help with the pain. There is some evidence to support their use, and they may also help with joint pain. There is no convincing evidence that steroids help with the skin manifestations of the disease, which rarely require treatment anyway. The more important question is whether steroids should be used to help treat kidney involvement in HSP. Children who develop renal complications (nephritic/nephrotic syndrome and/ or reduced renal function) are likely to have a poorer prognosis and recurrence of disease. Hence, debate and controversy continue on the role of treatment with steroids and other agents early in disease to prevent long-term renal complications. Corticosteroids, unfortunately, have not been shown to prevent the development of HSP-associated delayed nephritis. Despite the lack of evidence, those with severe renal disease are likely to be treated more aggressively due to the potential for adverse long-term consequences. Other agents used may include immunosuppressants such as cyclophosphamide, azathioprine or ciclosporin. This will normally involve the input of a paediatric nephrologist.

Learning Tip

Consider the following four models of the presentation of disease:

- Common condition with common symptom
- Common condition with rare symptom
- Rare condition with common symptom
- Rare condition with rare symptom

A myocardial infarction (MI) presenting with chest pain (common symptom) is likely to be more readily diagnosed compared with an MI presenting as indigestion (uncommon symptom). A rarer condition such as HSP presenting with the tell-tale rash as discussed above is likely to be easily recognized. The rare condition with a rare symptom is the trickiest and was discussed in Case 2. In reality, conditions present with a melee of symptoms, and teasing out the relevant ones is the real challenge. However, keeping the above classification in mind can help with the uncertainty one faces when making a diagnosis.

AKT PREPARATION

Options for questions 86–90:

a. Vitamin A
b. Vitamin D
c. Vitamin B_1
d. Vitamin B_2
e. Niacin
f. Vitamin C
g. Zinc
h. Selenium
i. Iron

Questions 86–90 refer to conditions that are caused by a deficiency in a particular mineral or vitamin. Choose the most appropriate answer from the list above. Each option may be used once, more than once or not at all.

86. Pellagra.

87. Beri beri.

88. Scurvy.

89. Which of the following statements regarding protein-energy malnutrition are true?

a. Protein-energy malnutrition is a problem of the developing world only.
b. Marasmus is caused primarily by a low calorific diet.
c. Marasmus is characterized by the presence of oedema in the infant.
d. Kwashiorkor tends to occur at the time when the child is weaned from breast milk.
e. Children with kwashiorkor are usually ravenous and have a very good appetite.

90. Late walker, obese with insatiable appetite and hyperphagia, poor suck as infant and low intelligence quotient. Which of the following syndromes best describes this child?

a. Angelman syndrome
b. Down's syndrome
c. Prader–Willi syndrome
d. Edwards syndrome
e. Rubella syndrome

BIBLIOGRAPHY

Barr DGD, Crofton PM, Goel KM. Disorders of bones, joints and connective tissue. In: Campbell AGM, McIntosh N. *Forfar & Arneil's Textbook of Pediatrics.* Churchill Livingstone; 1998. P. 1544–615.

Brown JK, Minns RA. Disorders of the central nervous system. Surgical paediatrics. In: Campbell AGM, McIntosh N. *Forfar & Arneil's Textbook of Pediatrics.* Churchill Livingstone; 1998. P. 641–846.

Di Vincenzo F, Ennas S, Pizzoferrato M et al. Henoch-Schönlein purpura following exposure to SARS-CoV2 vaccine or infection: A systematic review and a case report. *Intern Emerg Med* 2024; **19**(1):13–37.

Gardner-Medwin JM, Dolezalova P, Cummins C et al. Incidence of Henoch-Schönlein purpura, Kawasaki disease, and rare vasculitides in children of different ethnic origins. *Lancet* 2002; **360**(9341):1197–202.

Gunay-Aygun M, Schwartz S, Heeger S et al. The changing purpose of Prader-Willi syndrome clinical diagnostic criteria and proposed revised criteria. *Pediatrics* 2001 Nov; **108**(5):E92.

Hendricks WM. Pellagra and Pellagralike dermatoses: Etiology, differential diagnosis, dermatopathology, and treatment. *Semin Dermatol* 1991 Dec; **10**(4):282–92.

Jauhola O, Ronkainen J, Koskimies O et al. Outcome of Henoch-Schönlein purpura 8 years after treatment with a placebo or prednisone at disease onset. *Pediatr Nephrol* 2012; **27**(6):933–9.

Mrusek S, Krüger M, Greiner P et al. Henoch-Schönlein purpura. *Lancet* 2004; **363**:1116.

Saulsbury FT. Clinical update: Henoch-Schönlein purpura. *Lancet* 2007; **369**:976–8.

Tizard EJ. Henoch-Schönlein purpura. *Arch Dis Child* 1999; **80**:380–83.

Tizard EJ, Hamilton-Ayres MJJ. Henoch-Schönlein purpura. *Arch Dis Child Pract Ed* 2008; **93**:1–8.

Watanabe T. Henoch-Schönlein purpura following influenza vaccinations during the pandemic of influenza A (H1N1). *Pediatr Nephrol* 2011; **26**(5):795–8.

Weaver LT. Nutrition. In: Campbell AGM, McIntosh N. *Forfar & Arneil's Textbook of Pediatrics.* Churchill Livingstone; 1998. P. 1179–230.

19

Case 19: Recurrent candida infection

A 32-year-old woman sees you to discuss her battle with recurring thrush. She has been to the surgery on four separate occasions in the last six months complaining of creamy cottage cheese-like discharge, vulvar itching and dyspareunia. Swabs were taken twice, which confirmed the presence of candida species on both occasions. No other organisms were found on microscopy. The other two times, she was treated empirically with topical antifungals. Each time, temporary relief was obtained with recurrence of symptoms a few weeks later. She is married with the same sexual partner for the last 10 years. She is on the combined oral contraceptive pill. She is concerned that she may be doing something wrong and wonders what steps she can take to stop the infection from recurring.

Which of the following statements regarding vulvovaginal candida are incorrect?

a. *Candida albicans* is responsible for the large majority of vaginal candida infections.
b. Isolation of candida from the vagina is always associated with symptomatic disease.
c. Recurrent vulvovaginal candidiasis is defined as four or more episodes in one year.
d. Poor female hygiene habits are strongly related to cases of recurring vaginal candidiasis.
e. Patient should be informed that recurrent candida infection is a sexually transmitted disease and their partner should be tested, even if asymptomatic.

DOI: 10.1201/9781003449737-20

ANSWER

b, d and e are incorrect

Although candida infection of the vagina is very common, affecting three out of four women at least once in their life, recurrent infection is thankfully less common. It is thought that 5–8% of women suffer from recurrent vaginal candidiasis, defined as four or more episodes in a year. *Candida albicans* is the most frequently isolated yeast strain from the vagina. Other species, found rarely, include *Candida glabrata, Candida tropicalis* and *Candida krusei. C glabrata* is of particular interest as it often causes recurrent vaginal candidiasis. Candida is thought to enter the vagina from the perianal area. Candida is a commensal organism, a fact borne out by the finding that most women will carry candida in their vagina at some point in their lives without any symptoms. A full understanding of what switches candida from a commensal to a vaginitis-causing pathogen is still sought, although vaginal anti-candida defence mechanisms are thought to play an important part.

Understanding of the factors that may contribute to recurrent vulvovaginal candidiasis is paramount if we are to maximize the chances of recovery in our troubled patient. Below are listed some of the factors that may contribute towards recurrent infection and what advice can be given to the patient.

CONTRACEPTION

The role of contraceptives in recurrent infection is somewhat controversial, as studies have borne out contradictory results. It would therefore be a reasonable approach to stop the oral contraceptive pill in our patient to see if this causes any reduction in the episodes of thrush. Increased carriage of yeast has also been found in women who have intra-uterine contraceptive devices or use contraceptive sponges, diaphragms and condoms. Although this does not translate into an increased risk of symptomatic disease, stopping these measures for some period of time may be a reasonable approach. The risk of falling pregnant needs to be weighed up against this. The patient should be made aware of the lack of definitive evidence with regard to this advice so she may make an informed decision. Interestingly, one study, in which 15 non-diabetic women were followed up for 6 years, showed that the long-acting injectable progestogen Depo-Provera, given at 150 mg doses every 12 weeks, prevented episodes of recurrence in some women (Dennerstein, 1986). If not contraindicated, and contraception is desired, this may be used as a substitute for the above methods of contraception.

DIABETES

Sugar is an important nutrient for candida species to thrive on (Van Ende et al., 2019). Candidal colonization is also more common in women with diabetes. If the diabetes is well controlled, the risk of developing symptomatic candidiasis does not seem to be increased. Diabetic patients are, however, more likely to colonize the resistant, recurrent disease-causing *C. glabrata*. A history should be taken from the patient, and if symptoms are suggestive, a test to rule out diabetes should be performed. Interestingly, "sugar binges" have been linked with symptomatic vaginal candidiasis in some non-diabetic women. The patient should be advised to cut down on sugary food and see if this makes any difference to the recurrence rate.

DISORDERS OF THE IMMUNE SYSTEM

Recurrent vulvovaginal candidiasis has been linked with cell-mediated immunity defect. The mechanism suggested may be a poor T cell response to candida antigen in recurrent cases. Patients should be advised of simple measures to boost their immune system, such as healthy eating and exercise, cessation of smoking and adequate sleep. If there is a suggestive sexual history, a HIV test should also be carried out. Despite being considered an AIDS-defining condition in the past, it is now well known that most women with recurrent disease are HIV negative.

ANTIBIOTIC USE

It is frequently observed that use of antibiotics is associated with an increased risk of developing symptomatic vulvovaginal candidiasis. This seems to be the case in women who already have asymptomatic colonization with candida. It is thought that antibiotics wipe out the lactobacillus population in the vagina. The lack of lactobacillus may contribute to a rise in vaginal pH, making it more prone to infections. However, the fact that some women may lack vaginal lactobacillus, yet maintain a normal vaginal pH, suggests that other mechanisms, such as competition between lactobacillus and yeasts for nutrients, may also be involved here. The role of live yogurts in reducing the risk of recurrence is far from clear. They may be recommended in addition to other treatments, as long as the patient is aware that there is no concrete evidence of their benefit.

SEXUAL BEHAVIOUR

Sexual behaviour may also contribute to developing recurrent, symptomatic candidiasis. There is evidence that receptive orogenital sexual practices are a risk factor for developing symptomatic candidiasis. Increased frequency of sex may also increase the risk of infection. Candida carriage is more common in uncircumcised men. Transmission from asymptomatic male partners seems unlikely. Poor female hygiene does not seem to be related to candidiasis. The patient should be advised to wear loose clothing and cotton underwear to allow plentiful ventilation, though the benefit of this seems to be unclear. Local allergens or hypersensitivity reactions, e.g., to piercings, may also damage vaginal defence mechanisms and contribute to an increased risk of transmission and infection. If suspected, they should be removed if possible.

OTHER FACTORS

Other factors that play a role in symptomatic disease, which may not be applicable to our patient, are pregnancy and genetics. Higher levels of oestrogens are thought to enhance the adherence of candida to the epithelial lining of the vagina (the same mechanism may be to blame in increased infections with oral contraceptives). A strong family history may suggest a genetic susceptibility to disease. At this stage, nothing can be done about this except to modify what can be modified from what has already been discussed and to try the regimes discussed next.

Acute infection may vary in its presentation, but symptoms include little or copious discharge, usually described as cottage cheese-like, pruritis, dyspareunia and vaginal soreness. Examination may reveal the typical discharge and erythema and swelling of the female genitalia. Despite the availability and frequent use of over the counter treatments, several studies have shown that patient self-diagnosis is generally unreliable, resulting in an over-use of treatment. The lack of a simple diagnostic test means that diagnosis is based on clinical presentation and microscopy with or without culture and pH testing.

TREATMENT

Acute infection responds well to topical or oral azoles. Topical azoles are available over the counter and are generally very effective and well tolerated. Single-dose therapy (e.g., vaginal clotrimazole 500 mg pessary, oral fluconazole 150 mg) is also effective and may be more acceptable to patients. Recurrent disease is more difficult to treat. Mycological culture should be obtained to identify the candida species responsible for the infection. C. albicans species that are resistant to azoles are thankfully rare. In recurrent disease, topical or oral azole therapy should be started and continued until the patient is symptom free. A repeat culture should be performed to confirm that infection has been cleared. Half of women will relapse if a maintenance regime is not started. Acceptable maintenance regimes include weekly 500 mg clotrimazole pessaries or 150 mg fluconazole or a daily regime of 100 mg ketoconazole. The last is associated with a poorer safety profile and hence, is rarely used. Unfortunately, a symptomatic relapse is seen in 50% of women within a short time of stopping treatment. A long-term cure, therefore, remains elusive. The usual route is to repeat six-monthly suppressive regimes. C. glabrata has a higher resistance to azole therapy, making its treatment particularly difficult. Vaginal boric acid (600 mg in a gelatine capsule), amphotericin B suppositories and topical flucytosine have shown some effect.

Learning Tip

It is not always possible to stick to evidence-based medicine (EBM) during decision making. Physicians will often rely on intuition during the diagnostic process and management plans for patients. Intuition, as a decision-making tool, is employed with greater ease as experience increases. Trainees and newly qualified doctors may feel the need to refer to guidelines and well-established treatment protocols for a greater sense of reassurance in their practice. However, this must be tempered with the knowledge that each individual case that we see is unique, and the universal principles of EBM may not always apply.

AKT PREPARATION

Options for questions 91–95:

a. Candidiasis
b. Bacterial vaginosis
c. Herpes simplex
d. Trichomoniasis
e. Contact dermatitis
f. Lichen planus
g. Human papilloma virus
h. Foreign body
i. Atrophic vaginitis

Questions 91–95 refer to women presenting with vulvovaginitis. Pick the most likely cause for each scenario from the list above. Each option may be used once, more than once or not at all.

91. A 48-year-old woman presents with chronic vulvovaginitis. Examination reveals sore-looking labia and introitus. Some white streaks in a fern-like pattern are seen. Mucosal biopsy reveals a band-like infiltrate of lymphocytes at the junction of the dermis and the epidermis.

92. A 22-year-old woman presents with a one-week history of increased yellow, frothy vaginal discharge, pruritis and dysuria. Examination of the discharge reveals a pH of 5.0 and presence of mobile microorganisms. She has had three different sexual partners in the last month.

93. A 60-year-old postmenopausal woman complains of vaginal dryness, dysuria, post-coital bleeding and dyspareunia. Examination reveals a thin erythematous mucosa with a narrow introitus.

94. Consider these statements regarding genital warts. Which statements are false?

    a. The large majority of visible genital warts are caused by human papillomavirus (HPV) types 6 and 11.
    b. HPV can only be transmitted during sex when the warts are visible.
    c. Podophyllotoxin and imiquimod cream are licensed for the treatment of ano-genital warts in non-pregnant women.
    d. Cryotherapy is contraindicated in the treatment of genital warts, as it may cause extensive spreading of the lesion.
    e. Latent HPV infection may become active in pregnancy, causing extensive lesions.

95. Which of the following does not reduce the risk of acquisition of primary genital herpes during pregnancy?

    a. Prophylactic topical acyclovir applied from 20 weeks onwards.
    b. Avoiding penetrative sex.
    c. Using condoms.
    d. Abstaining from sexual intercourse.
    e. Avoiding oral–genital contact.

BIBLIOGRAPHY

Bachmann GA, Nevadunsky NS. Diagnosis and treatment of atrophic vaginitis. *Am Fam Physician* 2000 May; **61**(10):3090–96.

Dennerstein GJ. Depo-Provera in the treatment of recurrent vulvovaginal candidiasis. *J Reprod Med* 1986 Sep; **31**(9):801–3.

Eckert LO. Acute vulvovaginitis. *N Engl J Med* 2006; **355**:1244–52.

Falcaro M, Castañon A, Ndlela B *et al*. The effects of the national HPV vaccination programme in England, UK, on cervical cancer and grade 3 cervical intraepithelial neoplasia incidence: A register-based observational study. *Lancet* 2021; **398**(10316):2084–92.

Fischer G, Bradford J. Persistent vaginitis. *BMJ* 2011; **343**:1169–73.

Katta R. Lichen planus. *Am Fam Physician* 2000 Jun; **61**(11):3319–24.

Linhares IM, Summers PR, Larsen B *et al*. Contemporary perspectives on vaginal pH and lactobacilli. *A J Obstet Gynecol* 2011 Feb; **204**:120–1.

Sobel JD. Vulvovaginal candidosis. *Lancet* 2007 Jun 9; **369**:1961–71.

Sobel JD, Wiesenfeld HC, Martens M *et al*. Maintenance fluconazole therapy for recurrent vulvovaginal candidiasis. *N Engl J Med* 2004; **351**:876–83.

Talaei Z, Sheikhbahaei S, Ostadi V *et al*. Recurrent vulvovaginal candidiasis: Could it be related to cell-mediated immunity defect in response to *Candida* antigen? *Int J Fertil Steril* 2017 Oct; **11**(3):134–41.

Van Ende M, Wijnants S, Van Dijck P. Sugar sensing and signaling in *Candida albicans* and *Candida glabrata*. *Front Microbiol* 2019 Jan 30; **10**:99.

20

Case 20: Polymyalgia rheumatica

Your next patient is a 55-year-old woman who is well known to all the clinical staff due to frequent attendances. You note that she presented to your colleague six months ago with right shoulder pain. She was referred to the local physiotherapist, who diagnosed her with subacromial-subdeltoid bursitis. She was discharged by the physiotherapy team after a short course of physiotherapy. She then presented to a different colleague a few months later with generalized fatigue and poor sleep. It was noted that she had been suffering from stress due to loss of her job. She was trialled on antidepressants but returned to clinic a few weeks later as she was unable to tolerate the medication. At this point, blood tests including full blood count (FBC), urea and electrolytes, vitamin D level and erythrocyte sedimentation rate (ESR) were organized. Other than a marginally low vitamin D level, her bloods were normal. She was prescribed vitamin D replacement for eight weeks. As she settles in her chair, she tells you that the vitamin D replacement made little difference. She complains of morning stiffness, bilateral shoulder pain, neck pain and thigh pain.

Which of the following is/are true?

a. ESR can be normal in a considerable proportion of patients with polymyalgia rheumatica (PMR).
b. The prevalence of PMR is affected by geographical distribution.
c. The subacromial-subdeltoid bursitis is likely to have been a manifestation of PMR in this patient.
d. The onset of symptoms in PMR is usually rapid and can occasionally present acutely overnight.
e. Rapid response to steroid treatment can help strengthen the case for a diagnosis of PMR.

ANSWER

All of the above are true

PMR, as a condition, encapsulates some of the challenges that a primary care physician faces on a daily basis. It is a condition that has a huge variety of symptoms (all of which may mimic other conditions), has no consistent presentation, relies on a diagnostic test that is not specific to the condition, and responds to treatment that would also alleviate symptoms of other conditions which may masquerade as PMR. Yet, it remains a condition that is almost exclusively diagnosed and managed in primary care in the UK (Helliwell et al., 2013). Classically, PMR develops fairly rapidly over a few days or even overnight, but the staccato presentation that is seen in the case above is not unusual in primary care.

PMR is an inflammatory condition that causes considerable pain and stiffness in the shoulder girdle. Other parts of the body that are often affected are the neck, proximal aspects of all limbs and the pelvic girdle. Generalized malaise and asthenia, insomnia, low-grade fever and weight loss may be just some of the symptoms that a patient can present with in the build-up to the eventual diagnosis. Having a high level of suspicion and a willingness to revisit and revise previous diagnostic conclusions is required to increase the chances of a correct diagnosis when faced with an atypical presentation.

Giant cell arteritis (GCA) is a form of vasculitis that is closely linked with PMR. It is present in approximately a fifth of PMR cases (Ramon et al., 2022) and presents a significant challenge to the clinician, as missing this diagnosis can have devastating consequences for the patient. GCA may be cranial or large vessel GCA, the latter being particularly difficult to diagnose due to presenting primarily with non-specific constitutional symptoms. Red flags to look out for are listed below.

Red flags in PMR patients include:

- Temporal headache, scalp tenderness, jaw claudication and visual disturbances are suggestive of cranial GCA
- Persistent fever in suspected PMR should raise the suspicion of GCA. Consider GCA when dealing with pyrexia of unknown origin (PUO)
- Signs of vascular insufficiency, e.g., bruits, murmurs, absence of peripheral pulses
- Erythema around temporal artery, pain on palpation, reduced pulsation and thickening of the artery

There are a number of different diagnostic criteria for PMR, but they all are similar in the sense that they require the suggestive symptoms associated with raised inflammatory markers and absence of symptoms suggesting an alternative diagnosis. ESR is the traditional inflammatory blood test used as a diagnostic marker. An ESR greater than 40 mm per h (30 mm per h in the Jones and Hazleman criteria) is considered positive. It may, however, not be raised in PMR, in which case the C-reactive protein (CRP) is usually elevated. It is unusual, but possible, that both the CRP and ESR may be normal. Although the reasons for why the inflammatory markers may be normal in what is essentially an inflammatory condition are not clear, it may represent subclinical disease or a more benign form of PMR. Although synovitis and bursitis are often seen in PMR (to the extent that some researchers believe PMR to be a disorder of synovial structures), ultrasound is not routinely used in the diagnostic process. However, where the diagnosis is not clear, it would be reasonable to use ultrasonography, and as such, it has been included in the American College of Rheumatology and European League Against Rheumatism classification criteria. Elevated plasma fibrinogen level is considered as accurate a marker for the presence of PMR as ESR and CRP (McCarthy et al., 2013), but its use in primary care seems to be limited.

Oral prednisolone remains the primary therapeutic option in the management of PMR. It can also be used as a means to confirm the diagnosis of PMR when it is doubtful based on the presentation and blood results. In such cases, caution needs to be exercised, as many conditions that mimic PMR may also respond to oral steroids. Most guidelines recommend a dose between 12.5 mg and 25 mg at initiation. Some authors have suggested 0.2 mg/kg as a useful guide to determine the correct starting dose for the patient. This dosage is likely to ensure that a large majority of patients are initiated on a prednisolone dose within the aforementioned range of 12.5–25 mg. The final starting dose can be adjusted according to individual risk factors of the patient (e.g., diabetes or osteoporotic risk factors). There seems to be a considerable degree of variability as to how the dose of prednisolone is tapered, but a suggested management is listed below.

75-KG WOMAN WITH PMR

1. Start on 15 mg prednisolone for four weeks
2. Reduce dose to 12.5 mg for four weeks
3. Reduce to 10 mg for four weeks
4. Reduce by 1 mg every four weeks until able to stop or maintenance dose found

Recovery for individual patients is varied, which probably explains why there are so many different tapering regimes used in practice. Each step of the management plan may be extended depending on the patient's response. It is not unusual for patients to continue steroids for two to three years or in some cases, stay on small doses permanently. ESR and CRP levels can be used to monitor the response to steroid treatment. However, symptoms rather than blood results should guide the steroid tapering regime. Bone and stomach protection should be prescribed in all cases. Intramuscular methylprednisolone injections can be considered in patients in whom oral therapy is not possible. Patients who fail to respond or relapse frequently can be referred to secondary care for consideration of immunosuppressive medication. A relapse should raise the suspicion of a possible missed diagnosis of GCA requiring higher doses of steroids, usually in the range of 40–60 mg per day.

> **Learning Tip**
>
> In primary care, it is not unusual to come across scenarios in which there is no clear pathway for referral. One may find oneself confronted by a set of symptoms or conditions that can be considered to be almost wholly managed in primary care. Presentations of tiredness (as those discussed in Case 14), chronic non-psychotic mental health issues such as depression and anxiety, and physical pain disorders such as fibromyalgia are just some examples of conditions where specialist input may help rule in and rule out disease, but the day-to-day management over the lifetime of the patient tends to take place primarily in the domain of primary care.

AKT PREPARATION

Options for questions 96–100:

a. Septic arthritis
b. Transient synovitis of the hip
c. Perthes disease
d. Developmental dysplasia of the hip
e. Slipped upper femoral epiphysis (SUFE)
f. Lyme arthritis
g. Non-accidental injury
h. Malignancy
i. Köhler's disease

Questions 96–100 refer to children presenting with limb pain. Choose the most appropriate answer from the list above. Each answer may be used once, more than once or not at all.

96. A seven-year-old boy presents with a one-year history of limp and leg pain on activity. X-ray of the hip reveals widening of the joint space and flattening of a sclerosed femoral head, suggesting early avascular necrosis of the femoral head.

97. A three-year-old girl presents with fever and inability to weight bear the preceding 48 hours. Blood tests reveal a raised ESR and CRP.

98. An 11-year-old boy presents with an acute onset of limb pain after a twisting injury in the playground. On examination, he finds it difficult to move the affected leg and holds it in an externally rotated position. He weighs 70 kg.

99. Which of the following statements regarding Duchenne muscular dystrophy (DMD) are true?

   a. DMD is inherited in an autosomal dominant fashion.
   b. DMD occurs exclusively in males.
   c. Diagnosis is clinical, with a positive Gower's sign confirming the diagnosis.
   d. Prognosis is good, with most males remaining independent till the fourth decade of their life.
   e. Creatine phosphokinase (CPK) estimation is rarely useful, as it is often normal in early stages of muscle destruction.

100. Which one of the following is NOT a major manifestation of the Jones criteria for the diagnosis of rheumatic fever?

   a. Carditis
   b. Polyarthritis
   c. Sydenham's chorea
   d. Erythema multiforme
   e. Subcutaneous nodules

BIBLIOGRAPHY

Caird MS, Flynn JM, Leung YL *et al*. Factors distinguishing septic arthritis from transient synovitis of the hip in children. A prospective study. *J Bone Joint Surg Am* 2006; **88**(6):1251–7.

Cimmino MA, Parodi M, Montecucco C, Caporali R. The correct prednisone starting dose in polymyalgia rheumatica is related to body weight but not to disease severity. *BMC Musculoskelet Disord* 2011; **12**:94.

Diagnosis and management of polymyalgia rheumatic. The Royal College of Physicians; Jun 2010. https://www.rcplondon.ac.uk/guidelines-policy/diagnosis-and-management-polymyalgia-rheumatica

Ferrier P, Bamatter F, David Klein D. Muscular dystrophy (Duchenne) in a girl with Turner's syndrome. *J Med Genet* 1965 Mar; **2**(1):38–46.

Gonzalez-Gay MA, Matteson EL, Castaneda S. Polymyalgia rheumatica. *Lancet* 2017; **390**:1700–12.

Grazioli-Gauthier L, Marcoli N, Vanini G *et al*. Giant cell arteritis among fevers of unknown origin (FUO): An atypical presentation. *Eur J Case Rep Intern Med* 2021; **8**(2):2254.

Helliwell T, Hider SL, Mallen CD. Polymyalgia rheumatica: Diagnosis, prescribing, and monitoring in general practice. *Br J Gen Pract* 2013 May; **63**(610):e361–66.

Helliwell T, Muller S, Hider SL *et al*. Challenges of diagnosing and managing polymyalgia rheumatica: A multi-methods study in UK general practice. *Br J Gen Pract* 2018 Nov; **68**(676):e783–93.

Manzo C, Milchert M. Polymyalgia rheumatica with normal values of both erythrocyte sedimentation rate and C-reactive protein concentration at the time of diagnosis: A four-point guidance. *Rheumatologia* 2018; **56**(1):1–2.

Martínez-Taboada M, Blanco R, Rodríguez-Valverde V. Polymyalgia rheumatica with normal erythrocyte sedimentation rate: Clinical aspects. *Clin Exp Rheumatol* 2000; **18**(4 Suppl 20):S34–7.

McCarthy EM, MacMullan PA, Al-Mudhaffer S *et al*. Plasma fibrinogen is an accurate marker of disease activity in patients with polymyalgia rheumatica. *Rheumatology (Oxford)* 2013 Mar; **52**(3):465–71.

Ramon A, Greigert H, Ornetti P *et al*. Predictive factors of giant cell arteritis in polymyalgia rheumatica patients. *J Clin Med* 2022 Dec; **11**(24):7412.

SECTION ②

ANSWERS TO AKT QUESTIONS

Answers

1.   e

This child is presenting with a typical history of migraine preceded by a visual aura. The headache is thought to be due to vasodilation and increased blood flow to the extracranial vessels. Corresponding vasoconstriction of various intracranial vessels produces the varied neurological features of migraine. A history of migraine in a close family member pretty much nails the diagnosis when the clinical presentation is typical of migraine. In such cases, when neurological examination is also normal, further investigation is rarely necessary. Occasionally, to quell parental anxiety, brain imaging may be required. In this case, where there is little doubt about the diagnosis, of the options listed, prophylactic medicine to prevent attacks is the most appropriate next step. Prophylactic agents include beta-blockers, pizotifen and the tricyclic antidepressant amitriptyline. Further investigations are warranted where the diagnosis is in doubt or abnormal neurology is elicited. Keeping a food diary can be extremely helpful in identifying potential triggers of migraine and hence, limiting attacks without medication. The combined oral contraceptive would be absolutely contraindicated in this case.

2.   a

The history of headache in this child sounds quite benign. Usually, it is the parents who are more concerned by the child occasionally mentioning that their head hurts. There are no worrying features in the history that would point towards serious pathology. A full neurological (including fundoscopy) examination should be performed. If everything appears normal, it is appropriate to suggest to the parents that this may be an ocular headache caused by a refraction error and the child should have an eye test. Whether refractive errors actually cause headaches is somewhat controversial. However, one study (Gil-Gouveia) found that adequate correction of refractive errors in children who suffered with headaches (and had refractive errors) resulted in improvement in symptoms in 72.5% of children, whilst 38% of children reported a complete remission of headache, touting the possibility of a causal link. The child should be encouraged to drink more water. At this point, if adequately reassured, the parents will ask you whether the headache is to do with the amount of video games the child plays. At this point. a "wise, non-committing nod" may just allow the parents to tell the child to take note that the doctor thinks that they should spend less time playing video games!

DOI: 10.1201/9781003449737-23

3. f

This history is suggestive of cluster headaches, a thankfully rare phenomenon in children. As the name suggests, the intense one-sided headaches occur in clusters over a certain period of time, usually lasting a few hours. Patients may present with extreme restlessness and intense headache, enough to cause some to bang their heads against the walls of the casualty department. Autonomic features such as redness, watering and swelling of the eye, sweating of the face and nasal blockage may occur. Simple analgesics are generally not effective but are usually given. This child will require brain imaging to rule out secondary causes of headache. However, in the first instance, the most appropriate step is to try to relieve the pain. Treatment options include 100% oxygen, methysergide, triptans and ergotamine (Majumdar et al.).

4. b and d are true

Hodgkin's lymphoma most commonly affects the cervical and supraclavicular glands, although mediastinal involvement may be seen in two-thirds of children with the disease. An increased risk is seen in children from higher socioeconomic groups. Diagnosis is made by taking a biopsy from the affected node, which may feel firm or rubbery. The cell that is affected in Hodgkin's disease is the Reed–Sternberg cell. Although a diagnosis of Hodgkin's lymphoma cannot be made in the absence of Reed–Sternberg cells, they are not pathognomic for the disease, as they may also be present in some non-Hodgkin lymphomas and Epstein–Barr virus infection. The Ann Arbor staging system is used to help stage the disease. Stage I denotes involvement of a single lymph node region, whereas stage IV represents diffuse involvement of extralymphatic organs or tissues. The staging may be suffixed with A or B. The suffix "B" denotes the presence of B symptoms (fever, night sweats or greater than 10% weight loss in the preceding six months) and is associated with a worse prognosis. The suffix "A" is designated in the absence of these symptoms. Occasionally, the suffix "X" may be used, which denotes a bulky tumour. Chemotherapy forms the mainstay of treatment, though radiotherapy is also needed at times.

5. a

Haemophilia A, also known as classical haemophilia, is amongst the commonest of the bleeding disorders and is caused by an absence or low levels of factor VIIIc. Haemophilia B, or Christmas disease, is caused by a deficiency of factor IX. The two conditions present in a similar fashion clinically. Both are X-linked recessive disorders, and a good family history enables a diagnosis to be made. Unexplained bruising and haemarthrosis, when the child is mobile, occasionally raise concerns regarding non-accidental injury. Von Willebrand's disease is caused by a deficiency in factor VIII VWF and is inherited in autosomal dominant fashion. Epistaxis can be a recurring problem in this condition. ITP is the commonest of the immune thrombocytopaenias, in which there is an increased destruction of platelets. Bernard–Soulier syndrome is a congenital disorder in which there is a failure of platelet production.

6. g

These are tough questions and are specifically designed to pick out the bright examination candidates. It is not uncommon to encounter the odd such question in the diploma of child health exam (DCH) that many primary care physicians may consider taking. Paediatric eponymous syndromes are many, and in most cases obscure, making it difficult to prepare for all eventual connotations such a question may take. In practical terms, knowledge of individual rare syndromes is rarely useful. The important point is that the physician is able to tell that something is wrong. The diagnostic process for such rare syndromes may take weeks to months as further symptoms and signs develop and the child is put through many investigations by paediatricians and specialist paediatricians. Low serum copper levels are a feature of Wilson's disease and Menkes syndrome (also known as Menkes kinky hair syndrome; the alternative name almost certainly giving away the answer too easily). In Wilson's disease, the primary damage (from build-up of copper, possibly due to a defective transporter responsible for removing copper from cells) is to the liver and the central nervous system, and it should be considered in any child with abnormal liver function tests. Neurological manifestations may include psychiatric symptoms or extrapyramidal signs such as rigidity or tremor.

7. c

This question is also meant to confuse and test the confidence of the candidate in what they have learnt. G6PD deficiency leads to reduced glutathione levels in red cells, making them prone to haemolysis. It is an X-linked disorder, and symptoms may vary from none to acute haemolysis requiring exchange transfusion in the neonate. Treatment is avoidance of stressors that may trigger haemolysis, such as dietary factors (e.g., fava beans), drugs (e.g., quinolones) or severe infections. It is the most common enzyme deficiency in the world. Von Gierke's disease is caused by a deficiency in glucose-6-phosphatase. It is a glycogen storage disorder. The lack of the enzyme leads to the cell's inability to convert glucose-6-phosphate to glucose. Alternative metabolic pathways convert the glucose precursor to lactic acid, the build-up of which is possibly responsible for the resultant retarded growth and osteoporosis. The glucose-6-phosphate may also be converted back into glycogen, the build-up of which in the liver causes hepatomegaly. It is a rare disorder.

8. a

McArdle syndrome is another glycogen storage disease, resulting in inefficient use of energy substrate in muscle due to muscle phosphorylase deficiency. Exercise results in cramp, which tends to settle with a period of rest. Creatine kinase levels may be elevated. It is generally a benign disorder and may not even be picked up until later in adult life when the individual takes up strenuous exercise. No specific treatment exists, but the patient should be advised to stop exercise on the onset of muscle cramps. Failure to do so may result in rhabdomyolysis, myoglobinuria and subsequent renal failure.

9.   a and c are true

Congenital heart disease is an umbrella term, encompassing a large number of cardiac defects of varying extent and severity. It can be divided into cyanotic and acyanotic lesions, with the latter associated with a greater number of early deaths due to the lack of circulating oxygenated blood. The cause may be environmental, genetic or multifactorial. Infections (e.g., congenital rubella syndrome) and drugs (e.g., lithium or alcohol) during pregnancy have been strongly linked with cardiac malformations. Ebstein's anomaly is a defect of the tricuspid valve and is very rare. A ventricular septal defect (VSD) is the commonest congenital heart lesion. In isolation, it does not cause cyanosis. Usually, VSDs are small and close spontaneously, mitigating the need for any surgery. However, if the VSD is large, increased pulmonary blood flow results in increased venous return to the left side of the heart, resulting in left atrial and ventricular enlargement. The right side of the heart may also enlarge as the left-to-right shunt increases, leading to increased blood flow into the pulmonary circulation and increased vascular resistance. It may take a few weeks for symptoms of a large VSD to develop, as the pulmonary resistance at birth is high, resulting in minimal shunting across the ventricular defect. The infant may present with dyspnoea, sweating when feeding, failure to thrive and recurrent respiratory infections. Dextrocardia does not automatically imply a defect in the heart anatomy. Tetralogy of Fallot is the commonest of the cyanotic congenital heart lesions. The "tetralogy" consists of a VSD, pulmonary stenosis, an aorta over-riding the ventricular septum and hypertrophy of the right ventricle. The presentation of Fallot's tetralogy depends largely on the extent and severity of the aforementioned abnormalities, primarily the degree of right ventricular outflow obstruction. Usually, the infant is not cyanosed at birth, and this develops later in life. In the most severe form of Fallot's tetralogy, pulmonary atresia with VSD, the infant will be cyanosed shortly after birth and may be completely dependent on a patent ductus arteriosus for survival.

10. b

Chest pain in the paediatric population is a common presenting symptom in general practice but is rarely serious. Musculoskeletal pain arising from ribs, muscles and other structures in the thoracic area is common. The usual concern is cardiac chest pain due to well-publicized campaigns concerning adults. Cardiac problems rarely cause chest pain in healthy children, though consideration must be given to arrhythmias, congenital heart problems and inflammatory (e.g., pericarditis) conditions. Pericarditis classically produces a sharp pain, which is worse with coughing, deep breathing and leaning forward. The child is usually not very well either. Tietze's syndrome is a caused by a single (most commonly second or third), swollen and painful costochondral junction (hence differing from costochondritis, which involves multiple costochondral junctions that are not swollen). The diagnosis is clinical, and the condition is self-limiting, settling over the course of a few weeks to months. The underlying cause is unclear, but a preceding viral infection may be responsible. Slipping rib syndrome is caused by a disruption in the fibrous tissue joining the 8th, 9th and 10th ribs. This may be through trauma or lifting, resulting in the costal cartilages impinging on the intercostal nerves. Pulling the lower costal cartilages forward reproduces the pain, allowing the diagnosis to be made. However, abdominal causes of the pain may need to be ruled out to ascertain diagnostic certainty. The pain may last many months. Texidor's twinge, or precordial catch syndrome, is common in children and adolescents. A sharp pain, of short duration, occurs mostly just under the left breast or nipple. The pain may be made worse with deep inspiration (though others find relief with a deep breath) and may occur a few times a day. It does not signify any underlying problem and may be due to an impinged intercostal nerve or even associated with anxiety. No treatment is required, and it tends to self-resolve (Ives et al.).

11. h

These blood results indicate overt hypothyroidism with a raised thyroid-stimulating hormone (TSH) and low T4 levels. This patient is above the age of 60 and has ischaemic heart disease, and therefore, a gradual up-titrating of levothyroxine dose is the preferable method. Blood tests should be repeated 8–12 weeks after the change in dose and the dose adjusted according to the results.

12. i

Since no other information is given in the stem question, one must presume that the patient is asymptomatic. The blood results indicate subclinical hyperthyroidism with a low TSH and normal peripheral thyroid hormone levels. In the absence of symptoms, the most appropriate next step would be to repeat the blood tests after an appropriate interval, such as 8–12 weeks. If the subsequent bloods show persistent subclinical hyperthyroidism, then it would be appropriate to organize some imaging of the thyroid gland. Depending on local guidelines, this may require referral to the local endocrinology service. Toxic multinodular goitre, a solitary adenoma or Graves' disease is a possible cause of the persistently suppressed TSH, and treatment with radioactive iodine or anti-thyroid drugs is likely to be supervised by the specialist team. A possible alteration to the question may show a suppressed TSH, normal T4 but high T3. This would be compatible with T3 thyrotoxicosis and is managed similarly to overt hyperthyroidism.

13. a

Like the patient in question 1, this patient has overt hypothyroidism. Since the patient is young with no medical history, there is no need to gradually increase the dose of levothyroxine. The patient should be weighed and started on 1.6 μg/kg of levothyroxine. Higher doses are rarely required, but fine tuning of the dose may be required on the subsequent blood test 8–12 weeks later. Levothyroxine doses greater than 2 μg/kg should prompt investigation into compliance, gut malabsorption or inappropriate simultaneous use with drugs affecting levothyroxine absorption. Levothyroxine should be taken in the morning, 30 minutes before breakfast or any caffeinated drink, as food and caffeine may affect the absorption of the drug.

14. c

The commonest cause of subclinical hyperthyroidism in young people is Graves' disease. Toxic multinodular goitre and solitary autonomous nodules become the more common causes of hyperthyroidism with advancing age. Genetic variations have been shown to cause variations in TSH levels, with low levels seen in some black individuals. Smoking has also been shown to result in lower TSH levels in healthy individuals. The structural homology between TSH and human chorionic gonadotropin (hCG) molecules and their receptors has been well documented. As a result, hCG release during early pregnancy increases the level of free thyroid hormones and suppresses TSH. Glucocorticoids, such as prednisolone and dexamethasone, suppress TSH secretion, resulting in a fall in its levels. Stopping the glucocorticoid results in an initial increase in TSH levels before they return to pre-treatment levels after 48 hours.

15. e

The BWPS is a tool used to help evaluate the likelihood of thyroid storm. Points are given for a rising temperature, degree of central nervous system (CNS) dysfunction, extent of tachycardia, presence of atrial fibrillation, degree of heart failure, gastrointestinal dysfunction (including jaundice) and the presence of a precipitating factor. Interestingly, the serum levels of the thyroid hormones do not have any correlation with the severity of the illness.

16. b

Obstetric cholestasis, also referred to as intrahepatic cholestasis of pregnancy, is a condition of pregnancy in which there is pruritis in the absence of a rash with deranged liver function tests. Pruritis affects the palms and soles in particular. It will normally occur in the latter half of pregnancy and resolve after delivery. The risk of harm to the mother is low. It is, however, associated with an increased risk of pre-term birth and fetal death. A raised serum bile acid concentration is important for the diagnosis. Ursodeoxycholic acid can help reduce plasma bile acid concentrations and pruritis.

17. i

This case is suggestive of primary biliary cholangitis (PBC). PBC is an autoimmune disease leading to slow but progressive destruction of the intrahepatic bile ducts and possible cirrhosis. It affects mainly women and is more common in the fifth decade of life. Although a large majority of patients are diagnosed when asymptomatic, approximately one in five patients will present with non-specific malaise and pruritis. In 5–10% of patients with PBC, there will be no detectable AMAs. Ursodeoxycholic acid can be used safely in pregnancy. Liver transplantation has improved survival rates in patients with PBC.

18. e

HELLP syndrome is characterized by **H**aemolysis, **E**levated **L**iver enzymes and **L**ow **P**latelets. The abnormalities seen on blood testing are suggested by the name. A raised blood pressure and proteinuria may be present in 85% of cases, suggesting an overlap with pre-eclampsia. Approximately 10% of women with pre-eclampsia will develop HELLP. Management is centred on expediting delivery, as liver damage can be accelerated, with potentially fatal consequences for the mother and child. Acute fatty liver of pregnancy, a rare but serious condition, should be considered as an alternative diagnosis.

19. a, c and d are true

Oedema is not necessarily required to diagnose pre-eclampsia, though it may often be present. It is characterized by hypertension and proteinuria of 300 mg or more over 24 hours. It is diagnosed after the 20th gestational week. Symptoms occurring within 48 hours of delivery would also meet the diagnostic criteria. The onset of seizures heralds eclampsia. Budd–Chiari syndrome involves an obstruction of the hepatic veins. Doppler ultrasound is used to aid diagnosis. The Swansea diagnostic criteria are used for the diagnosis of acute fatty liver of pregnancy.

20. a

Vertical transmission is the most common mode of HBV transmission in endemic areas. HBV viral load plays a crucial part in the risk of vertical transmission. If the viral load is high, the risk of transmission may be as high as 90%. Transmission may occur through breastfeeding also. The mode of delivery, vaginal or caesarean, does not affect the risk of transmission. The risk of transmission can be reduced by giving the infant hepatitis B immunoglobulin within 12 hours of birth. Three doses of HBV vaccine should then be administered in the first six months of life. The use of antiviral treatment in the final trimester to reduce the risk of transmission is controversial due to concerns regarding viral resistance. Though the risk of vertical transmission of HCV is low, it is increased if the mother also suffers from HIV.

21. f

Endophthalmitis is a bacterial or fungal infection of the aqueous or vitreous humour of the eye. In most cases, it is caused exogenously by trauma or surgery of the eye. It may complicate 0.1% of cataract surgeries. It can also be caused by endogenous spread of infection from other parts of the body. The presentation is as in the case, with a painful red eye and reduced vision, and occurs usually a week after an operation. A hypopyon is the accumulation of white cells in the anterior chamber of the eye and presents as a milky white fluid visible in the anterior of the eye. Patients will normally be advised to return to eye casualty by the operating team if they experience such symptoms after an operation. Diagnosis is usually a clinical one and requires a fluid aspirate from the aqueous and vitreous humours for the purposes of culture. Loss of eyesight is a real risk if not identified early, and endophthalmitis is, therefore, considered an ophthalmological emergency. Treatment involves antibiotics, which are directly injected into the eye. Oral and topical antibiotics may be used in conjunction with the intraocular treatment.

22. a

These symptoms are suggestive of acute angle closure glaucoma (AACG). This is an ophthalmological emergency precipitated by an acute increase in the intraocular pressure due to failure of the normal drainage mechanism of the aqueous humour. The rapid rise in pressure results in pain, reduced visual acuity and headache and can induce nausea and vomiting. If left untreated, it may damage the optic nerve and cause blindness. Tricyclic antidepressants such as amitriptyline have anticholinergic effects and can trigger AACG. Patients may complain of preceding symptoms of halo around lights and intermittent blurred vision caused by intermittent closure of the angle between the iris and the cornea in the anterior chamber. These symptoms may have resolved on lying down and sleeping, as lying flat can relieve some pressure off the angle (this should be encouraged in an acute attack). Management involves the use of intravenous acetazolamide, which blocks the production of aqueous humour. Topical pilocarpine and beta-blockers are also used. Iridectomy is the surgical treatment of choice.

23. e

Conjunctival chemosis, though unsightly, is benign and usually self-resolving. In severe cases, the fluid-filled swelling can be bad enough to prevent closure of the eye. Treatment is with topical and oral antihistamines.

Red flags in the acute presentation of a red eye include reduced vision, moderate to severe pain, pain on moving the eye, photophobia, abnormal or painful pupillary reactions, hyphaema, hypopyon and uptake of fluorescein on the cornea. Differentiating between conditions such as anterior uveitis (inflammation of the iris and/or anterior ciliary body), scleritis and glaucoma is not possible in primary care, but they will present with varying combinations of the above red flags, which should trigger an ophthalmology referral.

24. a and c are false

As the name suggests, eczema herpeticum is mostly caused by *Herpes simplex virus* type I or II and is a potentially fatal complication of atopic eczema in children. Its alternative name, Kaposi's varicelliform eruption, was coined on Kaposi's observations that it looked rather like a chickenpox infection. Other viruses, such as coxsackie, may also be the underlying cause of the sudden eruption. The child usually presents with fever and systemic unwellness. Glands may be swollen, and a blistery rash is seen in areas of eczematous skin. New blisters continue to appear over a period of 7–10 days whilst old ones crust over. Superinfection with bacteria is not uncommon and can complicate treatment. Eczema herpeticum should be considered a dermatological emergency, necessitating referral of the child to specialist paediatric dermatology services. Oral or intravenous antiviral treatment is used depending on response and the general condition of the child. Recurrences in children are rare (Liddle). Preceding treatment of topical steroids is unlikely to be a causative factor. Eczema herpeticum may also be a complication in other conditions in which the skin barrier is faulty (David et al.).

25. All are correct

A cholesteatoma is essentially an abnormal growth of keratinized squamous epithelium, which extends into the middle ear and mastoid space. The term is somewhat of a misnomer, as there are no fat cells present in a cholesteatoma. The abnormal growth takes the form of a cyst and starts to erode into nearby important structures. Initially, it may present as an episode of otitis media with otorrhoea, which may be foul smelling. This may be associated with conductive hearing loss if the adjacent ossicles are affected. The GP may treat this with antibiotics, but the patient may continue to intermittently present with ear discharge. The onset of pain may be suggestive of extension into the intracranial space and may cause complications such as meningitis and abscesses. Mastoid involvement may lead to mastoiditis. The presence of vertigo indicates erosion into the inner ear and involvement of the vestibular mechanism. Facial weakness may be caused by the cyst impinging on the facial nerve as it transverses the middle ear and mastoid region. If suspected, referral to ENT is imperative. Investigations include audiometry to assess hearing and computed tomography (CT) and magnetic resonance imaging (MRI) scanning to assess the extent of the abnormal spread. Surgery remains the mainstay of treatment due to the potential for severe complications.

26. f

Angelman syndrome is a rare condition associated with epilepsy, severe learning disabilities and speech difficulties. The child's stiff puppet-like gait and vertical ataxia resulted in this being known as "happy puppet syndrome". Facial features include prognathism (bulging out of the mandible), tongue protrusion and a hooked nose. The child is noted to have a happy demeanour with sudden outbursts of laughter, resulting in a delay in diagnosis until such behaviours become apparent. West syndrome is part of a distinctive group of epilepsy syndromes termed "malignant epileptic syndromes". They are remarkably resistant to antiepileptic treatment and have a high seizure frequency. Cognition may be impaired, and a progressive dementia may develop.

27. e

Benign Rolandic epilepsy is amongst the commonest types of epilepsy in children. The child usually presents with the described abnormal neurology upon waking. The speech can be affected if seizure activity affects the throat. Drooling may be present. Seizure activity may progress to cause tonic–clonic seizures of the face and limbs on the same side. Occasionally, the seizure may become generalized, resulting in loss of consciousness and post-ictal confusion. An EEG may show centrotemporal spikes, a feature that is usually associated with a more favourable prognosis. Overall, in most children, seizures will settle by the time the child reaches puberty. If seizures are frequent, antiepileptic medication may be prescribed. Carbamazepine, levetricetam and sodium valproate are effective available options.

28. b

Breath-holding attacks are a benign, non-harmful "funny turn" usually triggered by emotional upset. Temper tantrums, pain from knocking oneself or excessive crying may trigger a short period of the child not breathing. This may result in the child looking pale and occasionally cyanosed. If normal breathing does not resume, the child may lose consciousness for a few seconds. Very rarely, it may result in a seizure. Reassurance of the parents is all that is needed, as most children will grow out of them before joining school. Pavus nocturnus, more commonly known as night terrors, is a sleep disorder that can run in families. The child may wake screaming and frightened with little or no recall of the cause afterwards.

Sandifer syndrome is a movement disorder associated with acid reflux in children. The reflux can result in paroxysmal spasms of the head, neck and back.

29. b is false

Retinoblastoma is the commonest primary eye tumour in children, accounting for approximately 3% of all childhood cancers. Although it is a life-threatening condition, prognosis is excellent, particularly when identified early, with 98% of children surviving the condition in the UK. However, recent campaigns have unfortunately displayed that there is usually a delay in diagnosis of retinoblastoma. This may be due to a lack of awareness of the presenting signs and symptoms of the condition in primary care or a low index of suspicion. Important signs and symptoms include an absence of the red reflex, an intermittent white pupillary reflex (leukocoria), strabismus, change in the colour of the iris, a worsening of vision, and unexplained redness and soreness of the eye. A delayed diagnosis increases the risk of extraocular disease and the need for more aggressive treatment. Recent advances in genetics have revealed a genetic form of retinoblastoma linked to mutations in the *RB1* gene. Children with this hereditary form of retinoblastoma are at increased risk of developing other forms of cancer later in life. These may occur anywhere in the body. Patients should be advised to avoid smoking and ultraviolet light (due to the risk of malignant melanoma). Extra care should be taken to avoid unnecessary irradiation from X-rays due to the increased risk of cancer.

30. a

Marfan's syndrome is a connective tissue disorder affecting primarily musculoskeletal, cardiovascular and ocular systems. Abnormally long limbs and increased flexibility of the joints are seen. Steinberg's sign is positive when the thumb, enclosed in the fist, protrudes beyond the medial border of the hand. Walker's sign is positive when the little finger and thumb overlap whilst encircling the contralateral wrist. Gower's sign is seen in Duchenne muscular dystrophy when the child uses their hands to climb up their legs whilst getting up. Rovsing's sign is seen in appendicitis where palpation of the left iliac fossa reproduces pain in the right iliac fossa, presumably due to peritoneal irritation. Scarf sign is elicited in the newborn and assesses the tone of the muscles in the upper limbs. Murphy's sign is seen in acute cholecystitis.

31. c

Pityriasis rosea is a benign, self-limiting rash of unknown aetiology. It is, not infrequently, seen with viral infections, leading many to postulate that the rash is of viral origin. It is commonly seen in children and young adults. Typically, the rash is preceded by a single scaly lesion, which may be round or oval in shape. This is known as a "herald patch" and can easily be confused with a patch of eczema or tinea corporis. A few days later, the widespread macular eruption appears, prompting a second (usually more worried) visit to the doctor. The child is usually well, and the rash is rarely itchy. Patients should be advised that the rash may be present for three months and treatment is neither necessary nor effective. Various treatment modalities, including antihistamines, topical steroids and oral antibiotics, have been tried but have failed to provide good evidence to support their routine use. Antihistamines, however, may be used if the child complains of itching associated with the rash. Important differential diagnoses include secondary syphilis, guttate psoriasis and cutaneous T-cell lymphoma. Pityriasis versicolor is a rash caused by malassezia, a yeast-like germ, and presents as pale or pink scaly patches primarily on the trunk, neck and arms.

32. g

Acrodermatitis enteropathica is a rare genetic disease inherited in an autosomal recessive pattern. It is likely that gene mutations result in a defective zinc transporter protein, resulting in reduced uptake from the intestine. This may become apparent when the child is weaned off breast milk due to low bioavailability of zinc in alternative milk sources and solids. Zinc deficiency may also be acquired in other conditions that cause malabsorption, such as cystic fibrosis. The rash is erythematous and crusted and may be well demarcated from normal skin. The rash can affect the eyes, mouth and nose, tips of fingers, knees and elbows. Hair loss may occur, and wound healing can be impaired. Superimposed bacterial and candidal infection may also occur. The genetic form requires lifelong zinc replacement, which results in rapid improvement in the child. Papular acrodermatitis of childhood is a papular eruption affecting the extremities, associated with anicteric hepatitis (raised alanine aminotransferase and normal bilirubin levels). It is thought to be of viral aetiology, with hepatitis B virus particularly implicated.

33. b

Molluscum contagiosum is a pox virus infection caused by direct skin contact. Sharing towels, baths or swimming pools with affected children may result in spread of the virus. Sexual transmission is the more likely route in the adolescent population. The lesions may become itchy due to surrounding eczema. Scratching can result in autoinoculation as the mollusca spread along the skin in the direction of the scratching finger, occasionally producing linear lesions. Parents should be reassured that treatment is not required and the lesions will eventually settle on their own, usually without scarring. Parents, however, occasionally insist on treatment, particularly if the lesions increase in number. A large-bore needle may be used to puncture the lesion. Alternatively, if the child is able to tolerate it, cryotherapy may be attempted.

34. a and d are true

Vascular naevi may be divided into haemangiomas and vascular malformations. Haemangiomas are benign proliferative tumours of endothelial cells, which are not usually present at birth. They usually appear following the first few weeks after birth. However, a pale patch may be noticed at birth at the site of their subsequent appearance. They are fast growing, with the bulk of growth occurring in the first six months of life. The rate of growth then slows down, and usually no signs of enlargement are seen after the first year of life. Over time they involute, and in the majority of cases they are fully resolved by the tenth birthday. Management is largely determined by their location. The vast majority of lesions do not require treatment and are managed by watchful waiting. There is a risk of them bleeding if caught, and usual haemostatic measures should be taken if this occurs. Haemangiomas in the nappy area may ulcerate and hence require special attention with frequent applications of barrier creams. Exposed lesions should be protected from the sun with high factor sun creams. Lesions around the eye (risk of amblyopia), mouth (feeding issues) and deep ones around the neck (tracheal compression) represent more serious manifestations, which usually require more aggressive forms of treatment. Treatment options include steroids, laser therapy, propranolol and surgery. Licensed for use as migraine prophylaxis, propranolol is thought to cause vasoconstriction in the haemangioma, encourage cell death and prevent further angiogenesis (Starkey et al.). Sturge–Weber syndrome is an association of a facial vascular malformation and a vascular malformation of the ipsilateral meninges and cerebral cortex. The capillary malformation occurs in the distribution of the first division of the trigeminal nerve. Vascular malformations by definition are fixed collections of dilated abnormal vessels (not proliferative like haemangiomas).

35. a

The canal of Schlemm is a circular canal responsible for draining the aqueous humour from the anterior chamber into the ciliary veins of the eye. Resistance to flow through the canal results in the build-up of pressure in the eye, leading to damage to the optic nerve. Congenital absence or abnormality of the canal (or any other congenital abnormality of the angle of the anterior chamber) can lead to primary buphthalmos or infantile glaucoma. The child will present with progressive enlargement of the eye as the intraocular pressure increases. The anterior chamber deepens, and a progressive myopia may develop. Oedema, inflammation, photophobia and epiphoria usually ensue. Delayed diagnosis will invariably result in damage to the optic nerve head, leading to an irreversible reduction in vision. Treatment is by surgery and involves a trabeculectomy to allow increased drainage in the angle of the anterior chamber.

36. h

Mumps is a notifiable disease and may present in a non-specific fashion, like other viral infections, with fever and malaise, resulting in the correct diagnosis not being made. The incubation period for mumps is between 14 and 21 days. Involvement of the parotid glands is what makes it easily recognizable, particularly when the swelling is impressive, resulting in the angle of the jaw becoming impalpable. The swelling may be unilateral to start with, progressing to become bilateral in the majority of cases. Mumps can affect any organ in the body, and hence, multiple symptoms may be seen. However, involvement of the CNS (aseptic meningitis), testicles (orchitis) and pancreas (pancreatitis) should certainly raise the suspicion of mumps, particularly if there is an appreciable swelling of the parotid glands. Diagnosis may be confirmed by demonstration of rise in antibody titres or direct culturing of the virus. Treatment is usually supportive and includes rest, plenty of fluids to keep the mouth moist and clean (as it may become dry as result of swelling of the salivary gland ducts), analgesia, and support and ice bags for painful testis. Boys (and their parents) should be reassured that sterility is rare, even after severe orchitis.

37. a

This child has hand, foot and mouth (HFM) disease, caused, in the majority of cases, by coxsackie virus A16. Other strains of coxsackie group A virus have also been implicated in outbreaks of the illness. The child is usually only mildly unwell, and the main concern may be the appearance of the vesicles or reluctance to eat and drink due to the lesions inside the mouth. Serious complications are extremely rare, and in most cases, all symptoms will have settled in a week. Due to the mild nature of the majority of cases, there is no need to keep the child off school. Getting HFM once does not preclude one from getting it again, as it can be caused by a number of different serotypes of enteroviruses.

38. d

This is the typical presentation of roseola infantum. Other names for this condition include sixth disease (a historical reference to the six rash-causing illnesses of childhood), exanthema subitum and three-day fever. The rash appears as the child improves in their condition, and most parents will tell you that they would not have come to see you had the rash not appeared. Parvovirus B19 causes slapped cheek syndrome, also known as fifth disease.

39. a, b and c are true

This question introduces the fascinating concept of the non-specific effects of vaccines. This refers to the holistic effect of the vaccine on the body, including on organisms not intended by the vaccine. It is no longer possible to look at vaccines simply modulating immunological response against the intended organism only. The way the vaccine interacts with the immune system is modulated by previous infections and immunizations. The Bacillus Calmette-Guerin (BCG) vaccine has been shown to reduce mortality from diseases other than tuberculosis by up to 25%. (Its hypothesized protective effect against Covid-19 seems to be debatable.) The sequence in which vaccines are given is also important. The increased mortality associated with DTP appears to be reversed by a subsequent dose of measles vaccine. A greater amount of research in this field is likely to yield a fascinating insight into how vaccines interplay with other organisms and the immune system. Option (d) is false, as maternal immunization with pertussis is currently being recommended between 28 and 38 weeks of pregnancy. Option (e) (known as the cocooning strategy) has been shown to be effective, albeit difficult to implement.

40. d

Vaccines may be live attenuated, inactivated, polysaccharide vaccines or genetically engineered. Attenuation of a live organism refers to weakening it in a laboratory before using it to stimulate active immunity in the recipient. Usually only one dose is required, as they stimulate a more effective immune response in the recipient. However, second doses are needed for some vaccinations (e.g., measles, mumps and rubella) where a sufficient response is not mounted in all individuals after the first dose. Inactivated vaccines require multiple doses, where the first dose merely primes the immune system, with an effective immune response mounted on subsequent doses. Oral polio vaccine (Sabin) is live, but in the UK, injectable polio (Salk) is used, which is inactivated. Rotavirus vaccine has been recently introduced into the routine immunization schedule in the UK, given at two and three months of age.

41. d

Ten per cent of the Applied Knowledge Test (AKT) for the RCGP exam is evidence-based medicine, which includes evidence interpretation and the critical appraisal skills needed to interpret research data. There is no better way to solidify one's statistical knowledge than by practising questions.

Conductive hearing loss has a prevalence of 10% in this population subset.

Of 100 people, 10 will have the hearing loss, and 90 will not.

	Disease positive	Disease negative
Test positive	6 (TP)	18 (FP)
Test negative	4 (FN)	72 (TN)

PPV = TP/TP + FP = 6/24 = 25%

42. i

There is not enough information given in this question to calculate the specificity of the test. The specificity of a test is its ability to correctly identify those who **do not** have the disease. This question is specifically involved with those patients who are already known to have prostate cancer. Eight hundred patients are known to have prostate cancer, and the test correctly identifies 780 (true positive) of them. It unfortunately fails to identify 20 of the patients who have the condition. These 20 patients would have had a false-negative result:

$$\text{Sensitivity} = TP/TP + FN = 780/800 = 97.5\%$$

In a real-life scenario, the test would have to be trialled on patients known not to have prostate cancer to determine its specificity.

43. h

This test has a sensitivity of 90%. There were 1000 people in the trial, of whom 100 had malaria (10% prevalence). Therefore, 900 did not have malaria. Of the 900 without disease, the test correctly identified 810. The specificity of the test, therefore, is 810/900 = 90%.

	Disease positive	Disease negative
Test positive	90 (TP)	90 (FP)
Test negative	10 (FN)	810 (TN)

NPV = TN/TN + FN = 810/820 = 99%

The positive predictive value of this test, incidentally, is exactly 50%, making a positive test in this scenario as useful as tossing a coin.

44. d is true

The *p-value* can be defined as the probability of getting a certain result. Research papers often quote their findings with the *p-value* as a tool to suggest that their findings are significant. Let us say there is a new treatment for tuberculosis. This new treatment (N) is compared against any old or existing treatment (O) in a trial. The null hypothesis (a hypothesis that can be nullified) is that treatment N is no better than treatment O. The hypothesis being tested will be the opposite of this, i.e., that treatment N is better than treatment O. The final results are that treatment N is twice as effective as treatment O in inducing a remission in tuberculosis. However, before any consideration can be given to this result, we must know if the result is statistically significant. Traditionally, researchers have used a *p-value* of 0.05 or less to suggest that the result is statistically significant. A *p-value* of 0.05 means that there is a 1 in 20 chance that the results obtained could have been obtained by chance; or in statistical terms, there is a 5% chance the null hypothesis will be rejected when it is true. A *p-value* of less than 0.05 is even more statistically significant, whereas the closer it gets to 1, the less statistically significant are the results. However, despite common usage, a *p-value* of 0.05 is an arbitrary cut-off, and by no means does a higher value suggest that the findings of the study should be automatically dismissed. It is for the researchers to set the acceptable level of statistical significance, which may be 1%, 5% or even 10%. The *p-value* is a test of statistical significance and has nothing to say about the clinical importance of the findings or the size of the effect. It merely informs us of the probability of getting the results by chance and therefore, the risk of incorrectly rejecting the null hypothesis when it is true (type I error) or incorrectly accepting the null hypothesis when it is actually false (type II error).

45. c is false

Cohort studies, cross-sectional studies and case–control studies are types of observational studies. They all have their advantages and disadvantages and are preferred over one another depending on the question being asked and the resources available. Randomized controlled trials are difficult and expensive to carry out when the condition or outcome being studied is rare. This can be overcome by using observational studies. A cohort study, also called a longitudinal study, looks at people over a period of time (often years). The most famous cohort study is perhaps the Doll and Hill study (1951), which followed up British doctors and linked smoking with increased mortality and lung cancer. Prospective cohort studies choose a cohort of people who do not have an outcome of interest (British doctors without lung cancer) and follow-up with them into the future whilst measuring any variables of interest (smoking). An external control cohort group can be assigned (British doctors who do not smoke) but is not necessary. An internal cohort group can be formed from the subjects who do not develop the outcome of interest. In some cases, all the data needed to make the comparison between two cohorts may already be available. In this case, a retrospective cohort study can be done, where the two cohorts are compared and data analysed to determine a relationship between the exposure and the outcome. Cohort studies are not ideal for studying rare outcomes. In this scenario, a case–control study is more useful, and this is discussed in later questions. Prospective cohort studies are prone to bias from loss of participants to follow-up, particularly if the outcome is rare. Retrospective cohort studies, on the other hand, can be affected by recall bias, as participants may recall past events incorrectly.

46. c

47. f

48. h

Questions 46–48 are looking at common ways of interpreting study results. It is important to be familiar with these concepts, not just for the exams, but to be able to usefully appraise clinical data and make decisions on best available data.

In the STEM question, we have the following data available:

- Absolute risk of developing disease in the control arm (ARc) = 500/100,000 = 0.005%

- Absolute risk of developing disease in the treatment arm (ARt) = 400/100,000 = 0.004%

The relative risk (RR) is just a ratio of the risk of an event in the exposure or treatment group to the risk of the same event in the non-exposure or non-treatment group. So, in formula terms:

$$RR = ARt/ARc = 0.004/0.005 = 0.8$$

The relative risk reduction (RRR) is the difference in the risk of the event (disease Q) between the two groups. It can be calculated as ARc − ARt/ARc; however, a simpler formula is:

$$RRR = 1 - RR = 1 - 0.8 = 0.2 \text{ or } 20\%$$

The absolute risk reduction (ARR) is the absolute difference between the risk of the event in the treatment and non-treatment groups. This is simply calculated as a difference between the two:

$$ARR = ARc - ARt = 0.005 - 0.004 = 0.001 \text{ or } 0.1\%$$

The number needed to treat (NNT) is a measure that allows us to assess the effectiveness of an intervention. The NNT is the average number of people who need to be treated for one person to benefit from that treatment. It is calculated as follows:

$$NNT = 1/ARR = 1/0.001 = 1000$$

49. c is true

This is an example where knowledge of these statistical and mathematical concepts is useful. In both trials, the RRR is 20%, which seems like a lot. But, the RRR is just a way of expressing the difference in risk between two cohorts. It gives us no idea of the scale of benefit in terms of actual numbers. In question 48, the NNT was 1000. In this question, we have the same drug treating a rarer condition but producing the same RRR of 20%. Let's see how this affects the ARR and the NNT. We have two bits of information available in this question:

$$ARc = 250/100,000 = 0.0025 \text{ or } 0.25\%$$

$$RRR = 20\% \text{ or } 0.2$$

$$\text{Since } RRR = 1 - RR$$

$$RR = 1 - RRR = 1 - 0.2 = 0.8$$

$$RR = ARt/ARc, \text{ so}$$

$$ARt = RR \times ARc = 0.8 \times 0.0025 = 0.002 \text{ or } 0.2\%$$

$$ARR = ARc - ARt = 0.0025 - 0.002 = 0.0005 \text{ or } 0.05\%$$

$$NNT = 1/ARR = 1/0.0005 = 2000$$

In this scenario, despite the fact that the trial showed the same RRR of 20%, the ARR was halved to 0.05%, resulting in a doubling of the NNT to 2000. This was all due to the fact that there were fewer cases in the control arm.

50. b is false

A case–control study is a type of observational study, like those looked at in the previous case. Two cohorts, one affected by the condition being studied (*E. coli*) and one unaffected by it, are compared side by side. Whereas a cohort study looks at the frequency of disease in exposed and non-exposed cohorts, a case–control study is interested in the frequency and amount of exposure in those with (cases) and without (controls) the disease in question (*E. coli*). An odds ratio (OR) measures the association between an exposure and an outcome; it does not imply causation, only correlation. We have three potential outcomes:

- OR >1 exposure associated with increased odds of outcome
- OR =1 exposure does not affect the odds of outcome
- OR <1 exposure associated with reduced odds of outcome

The odds are defined as the probability of an event happening divided by the probability of it not happening; the odds of throwing a 1 in a 6-sided dice is 1/5 (as opposed to 1/6, which is the probability). Now, back to the question at hand.

In our case group we have

- 45 people: 35 exposed and 10 non-exposed

In our control group we have

- 180 people: 60 exposed and 120 non-exposed

This data can be presented in tabular form as follows:

	Cases	Controls
Exposure positive	35 (A)	60 (B)
Exposure negative	10 (C)	120 (D)

Bearing in mind the aforementioned definition of odds, the odds of exposure in the case group is 35/10 and the odds in the control group 60/120. Since the OR is just a ratio of the two odds, it can be expressed as follows:

$$35/10 \text{ divided by } 60/120 \text{ or } 35 \times 120/10 \times 60 \text{ } (A \times D/B \times C) = 7$$

So, eating at the staff canteen (exposure) is associated with 7× greater odds of developing *E. coli*.

51. d

Haematocolpos is a rare condition caused by the onset of menstruation with an imperforate hymen. Blood accumulates in the vagina and may eventually cause swelling of the uterus and even the fallopian tubes. This may manifest itself as a mass that may extend into the pelvis and be felt transabdominally. Urinary hesitancy and frequency due to pressure from the mass may follow. Dissection of the membrane under general anaesthetic results in a release of the collected blood and subsequent relief from the symptoms. Wilkie's syndrome is a rare syndrome that may cause acute or chronic abdominal pain in children and adults. The third part of the duodenum is compressed between the superior mesenteric artery and the aorta, resulting in symptoms of upper gastrointestinal obstruction.

52. a

Intussusception refers to the herniation of the intestine into itself. Part of the bowel serves as the apex from where the herniation begins. The exact cause is unknown, but it has been linked with viral infections. The virus causes inflammation of lymphoid tissue in the bowel (Peyer's patch). The swollen, enlarged part of the bowel then invaginates into the colon for a variable distance, presenting itself at the anus in the most severe of cases. Since it is commonest in infants between the ages of three and nine months, the change in bowel flora as a result of weaning may have a causative role. Ultimately, pressure of the herniated bowel against the wall of normal bowel causes colicky abdominal pain, which worsens as the condition progresses. Vomiting commonly follows. Redcurrant jelly stool is frequently associated with intussusceptions and is stool mixed with mucus and blood. Treatment involves attempting to reduce the herniating bowel by means of passing an air enema. Surgery is required if this fails.

53. c

Pyloric stenosis usually presents in the first few weeks of life as parents report an increasing frequency of vomiting. A congenitally thickened pylorus results in obstruction of outflow of stomach contents. As the condition progresses, projectile vomiting follows, as the vomit no longer trickles down the front of the infant but rather, shoots over the shoulder of the anxious parent. The vomitus may become progressively blood stained due to the resulting gastritis. The infant usually feels hungry after vomiting and is keen to feed again. Traditionally, the diagnosis is made during examination of the child after a test feed. The physician is able to feel the olive-shaped mass in the right hypochondrium. Peristalsis may be visible as the surrounding muscles contract to push the feed beyond the narrowing. The loss of gastric acid as a result of vomiting leads to hypochloraemia, alkalosis and hypokalaemia. However, pyloric stenosis is usually diagnosed before the classical biochemical hallmarks develop due to early suspicion and use of ultrasound scanning (Hulka et al.). Treatment involves a pyloromyotomy, which may be performed laparoscopically.

54. a and c are true

Male infant circumcision can be an emotive topic. For some, it is a religious right and duty, the practice of which goes back thousands of years. For others, it is an assault on a non-consenting child and a breach of their human rights. This question, thankfully, is more about objective scientific evidence regarding the benefits and harms of circumcision rather than the ethical and moral dilemmas surrounding it. The overall consensus of scientific evidence seems to be towards greater health benefits compared with the small risks associated with the procedure. Indeed, the American Academy of Paediatrics (AAP) issued an update on their circumcision policy stating that the increased health benefits warranted third-party payment for the procedure. This was received with some stiff opposition, mainly from various European medical associations. The AAP does not, however, recommend routine male infant circumcisions, leaving the decision mainly with the parents. Health benefits include a reduced risk of developing HIV in areas of high HIV prevalence, such as Africa. Circumcision is also likely to be protective against syphilis, HPV and genital herpes. A reduced risk of chlamydia and gonorrhoea has not been demonstrated. The abrasion- and micro-tear-prone inner surface of the foreskin may be responsible for the increased risk of developing sexually transmitted infections. Circumcision is not associated with an increased risk of cervical cancer in the partner. On the contrary, it may be protective against its development. The risk of penile cancer is reduced with circumcision. Measuring sexual satisfaction, sensitivity and function is difficult; however, the literature does not suggest that circumcised males are at any disadvantage in these departments! Any such suggestions may be extrapolations of studies done on men who were circumcised as adults, in whom reduced masturbatory pleasure and increased threshold for light touch sensitivity has been demonstrated.

55. b

Wilms' tumour accounts for the majority of kidney tumours in the paediatric age group. It may present as part of a syndrome that includes aniridia (lack of iris), genitourinary abnormalities and mental retardation (WAGR syndrome). A deletion on chromosome 11 of a tumour suppressor gene, resulting in a loss of heterozygosity, is thought to be involved in the development of Wilms' tumour. Other syndromes with which Wilms' tumour has been associated with include Denys–Drash syndrome (pseudohermaphroditism and renal failure) and Beckwith–Wiedemann syndrome (macroglossia, organomegaly and macrosomia). It may be picked up as an asymptomatic abdominal mass in some children. Pain, non-specific malaise and haematuria may be the presenting symptoms in up to a third of children.

56. b

Syphilis is known as the "great imitator" due to the great variety of its clinical manifestations. It is caused by the spirochaete *Treponema pallidum*. Its clinical manifestations may be divided into primary, secondary, latent (early and late) and tertiary syphilis. This woman has presented with a chancre, a painless ulcer that is associated with primary syphilis. This will usually appear in the first three months of infection and may be associated with a non-specific illness. As the ulcer will normally self-resolve, it may be ignored, hence delaying diagnosis. Secondary syphilis is the most contagious phase and lasts for one to six months after the initial infection. The infected patient is most contagious during the primary and secondary stages. Tertiary syphilis will normally occur between 3 and 10 years after the initial infection but may present up to 50 years after the initial infection. A single injection of long-acting benzathine penicillin G is the treatment of choice in primary syphilis. Alternative regimes include azithromycin (2 g orally as single dose), amongst others.

57. h

Gonorrhoea is caused by the gram negative diplococcus *Neisseria gonorrhoeae*. An altered vaginal discharge may be present in up to 50% of women. Endocervical infection is frequently asymptomatic. Other sites that may get infected include the urethra (causing dysuria), pharynx, rectum and conjunctiva. One g of ceftriaxone intramuscularly is the treatment of choice if the susceptibility is not known before treatment. Previously, a combination of ceftriaxone and azithromycin was the treatment of choice, but this is no longer recommended. Patients should avoid sexual intercourse for seven days after treatment.

58. c

Chlamydia is caused by *Chlamydia trachomatis*. it is a very common sexually transmitted infection and may be asymptomatic in 70% of women. Of the regimes listed, doxycycline at a dose of 100 mg twice a day for seven days is the most appropriate. If the patient is pregnant or breastfeeding, then erythromycin 500 mg four times a day for seven days (or twice a day for 14 days) may be a more suitable option. Doxycycline is contraindicated in pregnancy. Azithromycin can be used if there is no suitable alternative. Sexual intercourse should be avoided until treatment is completed or until seven days after treatment if a single dose of azithromycin is used.

59. a, c and d are true

Neonatal herpes infection is a rare but serious systemic infection associated with high rates of mortality and morbidity. Clinically, it may present in three different forms:

- Lesions limited to skin, eyes and mucosa. This accounts for approximately 45% of neonatal infections. Intravenous acyclovir is required, and the long-term developmental outcome is good. If treated sub-optimally, it can potentially progress to more severe disease. Cutaneous disease may recur during childhood, requiring recurrent courses of suppressive therapy.
- CNS disease accounts for 30% of cases of neonatal HSV. This may present with non-specific symptoms of CNS disease such as lethargy and poor feeding. Seizures may also be a feature, and cutaneous lesions may or may not be present. CNS HSV-2 infection is associated with a greater morbidity. These children have high rates of developmental problems.
- The highest fatality rate is associated with disseminated disease, which accounts for 25% of clinical manifestations. There is multi-organ involvement. Although intravenous acyclovir therapy reduces mortality rates, the risk of death remains high at 30%.

60. a, c and e are true

In the UK, where safe feeding alternatives are available, HIV-positive women are advised not to breastfeed. Pre-antiretroviral therapy data suggests that women who are HIV positive who breastfeed increase the risk of mother to child transmission from approximately 14% to 28%. Midwives should have a sufficient understanding of HIV and mother to child transmission to enable them to include HIV antibody testing early in the pregnancy at the routine booking investigations. In the absence of interventions, over 80% of transmissions occur late in the third trimester, during labour and at delivery. However, about 2% of transmissions occur in the first and second trimesters in the absence of interventions. Statement (c) is true. However, if the mother is on antiretroviral therapy and has an undetectable viral load, the benefit of caesarean section is uncertain. For the newborn child, polymerase chain reaction (PCR) techniques are used for diagnosis of infections, as antibodies cross the placenta, making them unreliable for diagnosis at birth. However, the presence of HIV antibody at 18 months confirms that the child is unaffected.

61. g

Myasthenia gravis (MG) is an autoimmune disorder characterized by weakness in muscles, which is worse after exercise and may settle with rest. The presentation of the illness is determined by the muscle groups that are primarily affected. The most common presentation involves the extraocular muscles, causing diplopia and ptosis, and is commonly referred to as ocular myasthenia. Involvement of the bulbar muscles may present as choking after food and dysarthria. Proximal, rather than distal, muscles are affected if the limbs are involved in generalized myasthenia. MG affecting the diaphragm and the intercostal muscles can precipitate a myasthenic crisis, which can be life threatening. Anti-acetylcholine receptor antibodies are present in most cases, though antibodies against other targets in the neuromuscular junction may also precipitate the condition in rare circumstances. Tumours of the thymus are also strongly associated with the development of MG. Treatment is primarily with oral anticholinesterases such as pyridostigmine (too much of which can trigger a cholinergic crisis). Other treatment options include immunosuppressants such as prednisolone and azathioprine and a thymectomy. Plasma exchange and intravenous immunoglobulins may be considered in resistant cases.

62. e

Bell's palsy is an acute, idiopathic weakness of one side of the face. The onset of Bell's palsy is usually fairly rapid, and one must be confident that an alternative cause is not the reason for unilateral facial weakness. In Bell's palsy, all the muscles on one side of the face are affected, classically presenting with facial droop and difficulty with various facial expressions such as closing the eye or smiling. The forehead muscles are also involved, the sparing of which should raise suspicions of an upper motor neurone lesion being responsible for the presentation. Other red flags include bilateral symptoms, gradual onset, asymmetry of the oropharynx or swelling around the ear (parotid tumour), vesicles in the ear or mouth (Ramsay Hunt syndrome) or involvement of other cranial nerves. If there are any doubts regarding the diagnosis in primary care, the patient should be referred for urgent ENT or neurology assessment. The prognosis for Bell's palsy is usually very good, with most patients making a full recovery within nine months. An ophthalmology opinion may be needed if the cornea remains exposed due to an inability to close the eyelid. Similarly, prolonged facial weakness beyond three months is likely to need an opinion from plastic surgery in case physiotherapy or facial reanimation surgery is needed. The mainstay of drug treatment is corticosteroids if the patient presents within 72 hours of developing symptoms. The evidence for adjuvant treatment with antivirals is weak, but it may have a benefit if the paralysis is complete.

63. f

Guillain–Barré syndrome (GBS) is a rare neurological condition. However, it is the commonest cause of flaccid paralysis. Patients will present with worsening polyradiculoneuropathy, usually starting in the lower limbs, which can progress to involve bulbar and respiratory muscles and cause autonomic dysfunction. The symptoms usually plateau over two to four weeks and then gradually subside, though patients can be left with permanent disability, and it may also cause death. There is usually a preceding infective illness, which triggers off an abnormal immune response in the patient. *Campylobacter jejuni* is the most commonly reported triggering factor, though non-infective causes such as surgery may also precipitate the illness. Treatment strategies include intravenous immunoglobulins, steroids and plasma exchange.

64. d

The latest guidelines in diabetes management encourage the early introduction of SGLT2 inhibitors in patients with chronic heart failure, high risk of CVD (QRISK3 score of >10%

in above 40 year olds) or those with established atherosclerotic cardiovascular disease. In recent years, SGLT2 inhibitors have also emerged as key agents to prevent the progression of chronic kidney disease. It appears that their renoprotective effects are brought about by reducing glomerular hypertension and thus, are independent of their effects on blood glucose levels.

65. b

SGLT2 inhibitor use has been linked with diabetic ketoacidosis (DKA_ even in euglycaemic patients. The safest option in primary care would be to let the patient complete the ketogenic diet to allow target weight loss and then start the SGLT2 inhibitor. Restarting the ketogenic diet, once stable on the SGLT2 inhibitor, should not take place without discussion with her diabetes team and clarification of the risks of developing DKA.

66. b

A deficiency in the B vitamins (particularly folate, riboflavin, B6 and B12) is associated with homocysteinemia. Elevated plasma homocysteine concentrations have been associated with adverse pregnancy outcomes such as placental abruptions, stillbirths, pre-term birth and low birth weight. Although homocysteine levels drop in pregnancy anyway, supplementation with folic acid in the latter trimesters has been associated with an enhanced reduction in levels. Elevated homocysteine levels have also been linked to high coffee intake and cigarette smoking. However, due to the lack of strong evidence to support their benefit, supplementation is not routinely recommended with any of the B vitamins (except folic acid).

67. a

Vitamin A is a fat-soluble vitamin that is present in many foods. Fish, organ meat (liver in particular), dairy products and eggs are natural sources of vitamin A. Carotenoids are pigments that give certain fruits and vegetables their colour. Some carotenoids can also be converted to vitamin A in the body. High doses of vitamin A early in pregnancy are potentially teratogenic. A dose of 700–800 µg of vitamin A per day should be sufficient in pregnancy. Doses of 3000 µg/day (10,000 IU/day) and more have been associated with birth defects in the infant. One study estimated that amongst women who took more than 10,000 IU/day, 1 in every 57 babies born with a birth defect was due to the high maternal intake of vitamin A. Women should be advised to avoid excessive consumption of foods rich in vitamin A in pregnancy.

68. f

Copper serves as an important cofactor to a number of enzymes. Levels of copper increase during pregnancy, possibly due to altered synthesis of ceruloplasmin, which is the major copper-binding protein in blood. Low levels of ceruloplasmin are associated with Wilson's disease, an inherited disorder of copper excess. Low copper in the maternal diet has been associated with embryonic death and gross structural abnormalities.

69. e

Periconceptual folic acid, up to 12 weeks' gestation, is recommended at a dose of 400 µg/day. This is associated with a reduced risk of neural tube defects and congenital heart and limb defects. It also seems to protect against the risk of some paediatric cancers, such as leukaemia, brain tumours and neuroblastoma. There have been some concerns regarding an increased rate of twin births associated with folic acid supplementation in pregnancy.

70. a and b are true

Zinc deficiency has been associated with prolonged labour, pre-eclampsia, and fetal growth restriction and death. Zinc supplementation in pregnancy has been associated with greater birth weight and head circumference. Smoking appears to increase the metabolic turnover of vitamin C, thereby increasing the requirements of smokers. High-dose vitamin C supplementation is not recommended. Vitamin D supplementation in pregnancy is associated with a reduced risk of type I diabetes in childhood. The Healthy Start multivitamin tablet recommended for pregnancy contains 70 mg of vitamin C, 10 µg of vitamin D and 400 µg of folic acid. The enhancement of iron absorption from vegetable meals (non-haem iron) is directly proportional to the quantity of ascorbic acid present.

71. f

This child seems to be having confusional arousals, which are a type of parasomnia. Parasomnias are a group of disorders that are characterized by a series of behavioural and complex motor events, which can occur just as one is falling asleep, during sleep or as one wakes up. They can occur during the non-rapid eye movement (NREM) or rapid eye movement (REM) phase of sleep. The behavioural, emotional and motor abnormalities that can occur during parasomnias can seem somewhat bizarre, a fact that is evident from the names of the conditions that are included in this group of sleep disorders. These include sleepwalking, sleep terrors, sleep-related eating disorder, sleep-related sexual abnormal behaviours, exploding head syndrome and sleep paralysis. Occasionally, parasomnias have been the attention of high-profile court cases. In 1987, a Canadian man by the name of Kenneth Parks drove 14 miles to the house of his in-laws and murdered his mother-in-law. His history of sleepwalking and assessment by medical specialists eventually resulted in him being acquitted. The confusional arousals in this child do not require any specific treatment, and he is likely to grow out of them as he gets older. Some children, however, may progress to develop sleepwalking.

72. c

This patient is suffering from narcolepsy, which is characterized by excessive daytime sleepiness and unpredictable bouts of suddenly falling asleep. The patient seems to have lost control over his ability to control sleeping and waking. The patient usually has unsettled sleep at night, which may be punctuated with excessive hallucinogenic dreaming, either just as they are falling asleep (hypnogogic hallucination) or just as they are waking up (hypnopompic hallucination). Narcolepsy is classified as type I or type II. This patient has type I narcolepsy due to these recent collapses he has had. This is known as cataplexy and is typified by a total loss of muscle control. This loss of muscle control can either be localized, leading to drooping of the eyes or abnormal speech, or in severe cases can lead to a total collapse with inability to move or speak. The patient stays conscious through the event. The exact cause of type I narcolepsy is not known, but it has been associated with low levels of a brain chemical called orexin, the measurement of which in the cerebrospinal fluid (CSF) forms part of the diagnostic criteria of the condition. Narcolepsy is part of a broader set of sleep disorders knowns as central disorders of hypersomnolence, which include, amongst other disorders, Kleine–Levin syndrome. Kleine–Levin syndrome is a rare disorder, which mainly affects teenage boys and along with recurring bouts of hypersomnolence can include cognitive and behavioural abnormalities, hyperphagia and hypersexuality.

73. g

This woman is suffering from restless leg syndrome (RLS), which is one of the sleep disorders termed sleep-related movement disorders. RLS is more common amongst the elderly and females. Although the exact cause is unknown, dopaminergic dysfunction and reduced CNS iron levels are thought to play a part in its development. The creeping crawling sensation deep within the limbs can cause considerable distress to patients and disruption to their sleep. Dopaminergic agents such as pramipexole and ropinirole can be used in the treatment of RLS. Other drugs that can be used are gabapentin, pregabalin and low-dose opioids. Augmentation (worsening of symptoms with use of the medication) is an unfortunate consequence of some of the therapeutic options available (particularly levodopa), making management more difficult the longer the symptoms go on. Other sleep-related movement disorders include periodic limb movement disorder (repetitive movements of limbs during sleep), sleep-related leg cramps and sleep-related bruxism, amongst others.

74.b is false

OSA is a reasonably common sleep-related breathing disorder. It is characterized by either a complete collapse of the muscle and tissues of the upper airway (causing apnoea due to total blockage of airflow) or a partial collapse (causing hypopnoea where airflow is reduced by more than 50%) during sleep. These apnoea/hypopnoea cycles progressively reduce airflow through the obstructed airways, resulting in increasing respiratory effort until the point where the patient is awakened. Patients will report poor-quality sleep and excessive daytime tiredness, whereas partners report loud snoring, frequent waking or near-waking, and episodes where breathing stops. Although polysomnography in a sleep clinic is often used for the diagnosis of OSA and other sleep disorders, it is not necessary. Many sleep clinics now offer at-home sleep testing for OSA, where the patient brings the equipment home with them and attaches it to themselves before they sleep. Continuous positive airway pressure (CPAP) remains the mainstay of treatment for OSA. Mandibular advancement devices can be used for patients who find it difficult to tolerate CPAP.

75. b

Polysomnography is carried out in sleep clinics to help diagnose the nature of the underlying sleep disorder. During polysomnography, brain waves, blood oxygen levels, eye movements, chest, abdomen and limb movements, breathing rate and heart rate can all be monitored. Polysomnography helped elucidate the difference between REM and NREM sleep in 1953. Eugene Aserinsky and Professor Nathaniel Kleitman, working from the University of Chicago, discovered that there were periods of sleep when the eyes would dart back and forth rapidly. This was associated with rather active brain waves, much like those present when awake. In true scientific fashion, they carried out further experiments on their own children, which seemed to replicate the results and led them to defining the two distinct phases of sleep. REM was further shown to be associated with the dream phase of sleep. Further studies eventually demonstrated the now well-understood cycling between REM and NREM through the night as the normal pattern of sleep.

76. e

This woman is likely to be suffering from drop attacks. An idiopathic drop attack is a fall to the floor, usually without warning, not resulting in a loss of consciousness. There is a sudden loss of muscular control of the limbs, which results in the fall. The underlying cause in the majority of cases remains unknown, and therefore, they are considered to be a functional neurological disorder. They occur more often in women and may be related to underlying psychological distress. An anxiety state may actually precede the drop attack. Injuries with the fall are not uncommon. Functional seizures may present in a similar fashion. Drop attacks are also not unusual amongst the elderly, and can be followed by prolonged periods of inability to get back up again, which can be hugely distressing and lead to rhabdomyolysis due to prolonged compression of the skeletal muscle.

77. g

Bowhunter's syndrome gets its name from the neck position that a bowman assumes whilst shooting an arrow. The rotational position of the neck results in occlusion of the vertebral artery, resulting in posterior circulation ischaemia. The resultant vertebrobasilar insufficiency results in symptoms of dizziness but can also cause vertigo. Since the left vertebral artery is more often the dominant of the two vertebral arteries, occlusion of it is more likely to produce significant syncopal symptoms when compressed. The most common cause of the compression is cervical spondylosis, though frequent chiropractic manipulation and subluxation of the cervical spine due to inflammatory arthritis have also been suggested as potential triggers. If left undiagnosed, it may cause permanent neurological damage.

78. c

Subclavian steal syndrome is another condition that results in vertebrobasilar insufficiency. This condition is characterized by a stenosis in the subclavian artery proximal to the origin of the vertebral artery. The vertebral arteries then combine to form the basilar artery, which constitutes the posterior circulation, supplying blood to the posterior portion of the brain, including the cerebellum, occipital lobes and the brainstem. Vigorous exercise, particularly involving the arm, results in an increased need for oxygen delivery, which the body tries to achieve by increasing blood flow to the arm. Due to the subclavian artery stenosis, blood is "stolen" from the ipsilateral vertebral artery, resulting in vertebrobasilar insufficiency and its associated symptoms. The arm pain and paraesthesia are caused by the restriction in blood flow to the arm. As the vertebrobasilar arterial system supplies blood to the vestibular and auditory systems, any condition causing a reduction in blood flow through it can cause neurotological symptoms such as vertigo.

79. e

Roflumilast is a phosphodiesterase type-4 inhibitor with anti-inflammatory properties. It can be used as an add on to bronchodilator therapy in patients with severe COPD, defined as having a forced expiratory volume in 1 second (FEV1) after a bronchodilator of less than 50%. The patient needs to have had two or more exacerbations in the previous 12 months despite triple therapy with LAMA/LABA/ICS combination. Roflumilast is a specialist-initiated medication. It is contraindicated in those with cancer, with a history of depression with suicidal ideation, on immunosuppressive drugs, or with moderate to severe heart failure. It must also not be initiated in the presence of severe acute infection.

80. c

Although all given options may be appropriate in the management of this patient, priority should be given to the principle of primum non nocere (first do no harm). Pioglitazone is contraindicated in heart failure and therefore should be stopped in this patient.

81. d

Sex-cord stromal tumours account for about 5% of ovarian tumours. Sertoli–Leydig cell tumours are a rare type of sex-cord stromal tumours. Patients may present with signs of virilization due to excessive testosterone production by the tumour. The tumour is usually benign and unilateral. Management is determined by the age of presentation stage and differentiation of the tumour.

82. e

Meigs syndrome is a rare disease complex consisting of a benign ovarian tumour (classically a fibroma), ascites and pleural effusion. The mechanism by which fluid collects in the peritoneal cavity and pleural space is unclear. However, removal of the tumour results in resolution of the fluid. Ascites and pleural effusion may also occur with ovarian malignancies.

83. a

Ovarian torsion occurs when the ovarian pedicle rotates on its long axis, cutting off venous and lymphatic drainage. Prolonged torsion can cause venous and arterial thrombosis, resulting in ovarian infarction. Pregnancy (due to laxity of supporting tissues) and ovulation induction (possibly due to enlarged ovaries as a result of multiple maturing follicles) increase the risk of torsion. The list of differential diagnoses is long, making diagnosis difficult, as any cause of an acute abdomen may mimic ovarian torsion. White cell count may be raised. Treatment may involve untwisting of the adnexa or surgical removal of the ovary.

84. d

The International Federation of Gynaecology and Obstetrics (FIGO) staging classifications are used to stage gynaecological cancers. Wells score and modified Wells score are used in the diagnosis of deep vein thrombosis and pulmonary embolus, respectively. The risk of malignancy index (RMI) 1 and 2 are used to determine the risk of malignancy in a pelvic mass. Scores based on ultrasound features, the woman's menopausal state and Ca-125 levels are used to determine the final score. The Melasma Area and Severity Index (MASI) is used to determine the severity of melasma. The nine most androgen-sensitive areas of the body are given a score of one to four, depending on the severity of hairiness. This is then used to calculate the Ferriman–Gallwey score. A score greater than 8 suggests hirsutism. The scoring system is subjective and does not take into account the degree to which the problem affects the patient.

85. b and c are true

Bilateral ovarian wedge resection was the first surgical treatment used to induce ovulation in women with PCOS. The introduction of agents such as clomifene resulted in the temporary abandonment of surgical methods. Laparoscopy revived the use of surgical methods, and currently, the most widely used technique is laparoscopic ovarian diathermy using electrocautery. Approximately four out of five women will ovulate after laparoscopic ovarian surgery (LOS), if they fail to respond to clomifene, and a half will fall pregnant. Although LOS does reduce the levels of circulating androgens, its role in the treatment of acne and hirsutism has not been looked at. LOS, however, does not improve insulin resistance or the above-mentioned lipoprotein abnormalities. Older surgical techniques have been associated with an increased risk of developing hypertension and diabetes later in life.

86. e

Deficiency in niacin (vitamin B_3) causes pellagra, which classically causes the triad of dementia, diarrhoea and dermatitis (Hendriks), the dermatitis being the most common manifestation in children. Niacin is a water-soluble vitamin and is derived from the diet and from the conversion of the amino acid tryptophan. Bioavailability is high in meat and fortified grains. The dermatitis of pellagra affects exposed areas such as the neck (Casals necklace: named after the Spanish physician who first described the rash in peasants), cheeks and the extremities and may mimic sunburn. It is common in parts of the world where the main food source is maize due the lack of bioavailability of niacin and tryptophan in maize. Other causes include use of the anti-tuberculosis drug isoniazid (which blocks tryptophan conversion to niacin), carcinoid tumour (which diverts tryptophan conversion to serotonin) and Hartnup disease (impaired tryptophan transport).

87. c

Infantile beri beri is caused by vitamin B1 (thiamine) deficiency and is associated with a predominantly polished rice diet (the outer layer, which is rich in the vitamin, is removed due to over-soaking or washing the rice). The thiamine-deficient Mum suckles the child with thiamine-deficient milk. The young infant may be irritable and drowsy in the early stages, only to later present with acute cardiac failure. Neurological manifestations of the disease include encephalopathy, seizures, coma and eventually death. Treatment is with parental thiamine administration. Resolution of the symptoms confirms the diagnosis.

88. f

Once the scourge of seafarers (earning it the name *the plague of the sea*), scurvy, a result of vitamin C deficiency, is now rare. Vitamin C plays important and varied functions in the body, and hence, the signs and symptoms of deficiency may also be wide and varied. Petechial skin haemorrhages, irritability and impaired growth may be early signs seen in childhood. Bleeding gums due to fragile capillaries may result in loosening of the newly erupting teeth. Bleeding may occur around bones, leading to painful swellings of the lower limbs. Treatment is with replacement.

Other manifestations of this exam question could have included xerophthalmia (vitamin A deficiency), rickets (vitamin D deficiency), acrodermatitis enteropathica (zinc deficiency) and Keshan disease (selenium deficiency).

89. b and d are true

Protein-energy malnutrition encompasses a number of conditions, of which kwashiorkor and marasmus are the best described. Marasmus is essentially caused by a low-calorific diet in which the child has access to very little of what is otherwise a nutritionally complete diet. The child is usually ravenous (unlike the child with kwashiorkor, who is listless, irritable and has a depressed appetite). Biochemical abnormalities are less common in marasmus in comparison to kwashiorkor. The child is thin with reduced weight and loss of fat and muscle tissue. Provision of ample calories results in the child regaining weight, and the prognosis is generally good when identified and treated in infancy. Kwashiorkor is caused by a deficiency in protein intake, which occurs as breast milk is eliminated from the diet. Low protein content of the weaned foods leads to a decrease in total energy intake and nutritional deficiencies. A concurrent increase in the risk of enteric infections from various bacteria worsens the nutritional deficiencies and increases the risk of death. Although more common in the developing world, protein-energy malnutrition is seen in the industrialized world in the context of neglect and fad diets.

90. c

These are all syndromes associated with mental retardation. Prader–Willi syndrome is an autosomal dominant genetic condition in which the child may be hypotonic with developmental delay and have behavioural issues, specifically concerning food. Obesity is common and may not be entirely down to over-eating, as minor endocrine abnormalities are likely to contribute to the problem. Hypogonadism is also a common feature. Genetic testing is required for the diagnosis. Angelman syndrome is also known as happy puppet syndrome. Rubella syndrome is caused by fetal infection with rubella in non-immune mothers in the first trimester. This is a particularly devastating infection, leading to a number of mental and physical handicaps including deafness, visual problems and microcephaly. Down's syndrome is also associated with obesity.

91. f

Lichen planus is an inflammatory condition of unknown cause, which may affect the skin, oral cavity, genitalia, hair and nails. On the skin, it will typically present as itchy, polygonal, flat-topped papules. The reticulated white streaks are known as Wickham striae. A punch biopsy of the rash will reveal the above-described histology. Steroids form the mainstay of treatment.

92. d

Trichomoniasis is a sexually transmitted disease caused by the intracellular parasite *Trichomonas vaginalis*. It is more common in women who have more than one sexual partner and who have sex twice or more in a week. Mobile trichomonads are seen on a wet mount. Treatment is with oral metronidazole or tinidazole.

93. i

Atrophic vaginitis is caused by a lack of oestrogen. A mild discharge may be associated with this. Therefore, infective causes of vaginitis should be ruled out. It may also be associated with urinary symptoms such as dysuria and urinary incontinence. Treatment is usually with topical hormone replacement therapy.

94. b and d are false

HPV is one of the most common causes of sexually transmitted infection worldwide. Over 200 types of the virus have been identified, but HPV types 6 and 11 are most frequently implicated in genital warts, whereas types 16 and 18 cause the majority of cases of cervical cancer. The virus can be transmitted in the absence of visible warts, and therefore, it is recommended to use a condom during intercourse. It can also be transmitted by skin to skin contact and the sharing of sex toys. The HPV vaccination programme in the UK has been very successful in reducing the transmission of the virus. The vaccine is offered to all boys and girls aged 12 to 13. Podophyllotoxin is an antimitotic that prevents the cells of the wart from dividing and increasing in number. Imiquimod works as an immune modulator, encouraging the immune system to attack the virus. Both are effective against genital warts and allow safe treatment at home.

95. a and b are correct

There is no evidence that prophylactic topical acyclovir reduces the risk of acquiring herpes infection. Similarly, avoiding penetrative sex in the absence of condoms may still transmit the virus, as skin to skin contact may be sufficient to pass on the virus. It may be advisable to abstain from sex in the third trimester, as acquisition in the third trimester is associated with the highest risk to the neonate.

96. c
97. a
98. e

Perthes disease is a self-limiting disorder in which there is ischaemia of the femoral head. It is more common in boys and usually has an insidious onset. As with all hip pathologies, the pain may be poorly localized, with the child complaining of knee or thigh pain. Destruction of the epiphyses (and sometimes of the adjacent metaphysis) interspersed with periods of reconstruction result in anatomical abnormalities of the femoral head and neck. Hip movements are reduced due to the anatomical abnormalities and protective muscle spasm. FBC, ESR and CRP are normal. Being able to correctly diagnose septic arthritis is of the utmost importance due to the potential for devastating joint destruction. Large joints are mainly affected. Distinguishing septic arthritis from transient synovitis of the hip can be quite challenging. The presence of fever, raised CRP, raised ESR, a raised serum white cell count and inability to weight bear all suggest septic arthritis (Caird et al.). The child is usually unwell. Slipped upper femoral epiphysis (SUFE) is commoner in boys who are obese and gonadally immature. Gradual slippage of the capital femoral epiphyses posteriorly and inferiorly results in pain, swelling and reduction in hip movements. This is usually a slow process. The boy in question 73 has developed acute SUFE in which the twisting injury has caused an acute slip of the capital femoral epiphyses. This may be amenable to reduction by gentle manipulation and pinning. Reduction in a chronic slip is avoided due to the potential for compromising the blood supply to the femoral head. Bone tumours can present with night pain or as pathological fractures. Köhler's disease is an osteochondrosis of the tarsal navicular bone and may present as a limp. Osteochondroses are a group of disorders that affect the growing skeleton at the ossification centres.

99. None of the above are true

DMD is the commonest of the muscular dystrophies and is inherited in X-linked recessive fashion. The term "muscular dystrophy" refers to a group of muscle disorders that are degenerative and inevitably progressive. The genetic defect in DMD affects the production of dystrophin, a protein that forms part of the cytoskeleton of muscle cells. DMD occurs *almost* exclusively in males, as it can occur in females with Turner syndrome (XO), where the protective effect of the second X chromosome is missing, allowing expression of the recessive allele on the affected sex chromosome (Ferrier et al.). The young child is usually slow to walk and has a tendency to fall often. Gower's sign describes the child getting up in a particular way, climbing up his legs due to weakness. This, however, is not specific to DMD and can occur due to any cause of muscle weakness. Most children will be in a wheelchair by their 12th birthday due to the devastating progression of the illness. Up to a third of children may have concomitant learning difficulties, which may be accounted for by the presence of dystrophin in neuronal cells also. Creatine phosphokinase (CPK) levels are hugely elevated early in disease. As the disease progresses and normal muscle is replaced by redundant tissue, the CPK levels will gradually drop and may not be too far off normal. Electromyography may be useful, but diagnosis is by muscle biopsy. Management revolves around maintaining independence for as long as is possible and meeting the child's social and psychological needs. Cardiorespiratory complications increase with time, and death usually occurs by the second decade of life.

100. d

A clear infective trigger is implicated in the development of acute rheumatic fever: the Lancefield group A β-haemolytic streptococcus. Diagnosis of acute rheumatic fever requires evidence of streptococcal infection (e.g., positive throat swab, history of scarlet fever, increased antistreptolysin-O titre) along with either two major or one major and two minor manifestations of the Jones criteria. Chronic cardiac disease is a serious complication of rheumatic fever, and the child may present with endocarditis, myocarditis or pericarditis in acute disease. A murmur on auscultation, tachycardia, bradycardia (due to partial heart block) and a pericardial friction rub all suggest cardiac involvement. In the most severe cases, the child may present with signs and symptoms of congestive cardiac failure. Polyarthritis may present as acutely swollen and inflamed joints or as vague joint aches and is characteristically flitting (moving around quickly) and fleeting (coming and going quickly). Larger joints are more commonly affected than smaller joints. Sydenham's chorea (also known as Saint Vitus dance) is a particularly troublesome clinical manifestation of rheumatic fever. It is well recognized that there are physical and psychological aspects to the involuntary movements, which are non-repetitive, irregular, and may be focal or generalized. Emotional stress may make the movements worse, and they tend to disappear once the child is asleep. Overall, the chorea may have a devastating impact on the child's functional capabilities. Firm, painless subcutaneous nodules are an uncommon clinical manifestation of rheumatic fever, affecting approximately 1 in 10 patients. They are usually combined with severe cardiac involvement. The rash associated with acute rheumatic fever is erythema marginatum. Occurring mostly on the limbs and trunk, it consists of erythematous rings with pale centres and varies in shape and site from hour to hour. Erythema multiforme consists of target lesions (red centre with surrounding pale area) and is commonly caused by infection or as a reaction to a drug.

Index

Page numbers in *italic* indicate figures and **bold** indicate tables, respectively.

Printed in the United States
by Baker & Taylor Publisher Services